Dissociation in Borderline Personality Disorder

Annegret Krause-Utz

Dissociation in Borderline Personality Disorder

Associations with Trauma and Neurobiology

palgrave
macmillan

Annegret Krause-Utz
Department of Clinical Psychology
Institute of Psychology
Leiden University
Leiden, Zuid-Holland
The Netherlands

ISBN 978-3-032-06338-0 ISBN 978-3-032-06339-7 (eBook)
https://doi.org/10.1007/978-3-032-06339-7

This Palgrave Macmillan imprint is published by the registered company Springer Nature Switzerland AG
The registered company address is: Gewerbestrasse 11, 6330 Cham, Switzerland

Acknowledgements I would like to thank Christian Schmahl and Brin Grenyer for the rich professional discussions about the topic and their input. Thank you to all participants and individuals with lived experience who contributed to the research described in this pivot. Thank you to all of my students and colleagues who raised important questions and stimulated reflections on this research. I would like to thank Olivia Gadberry for proof-reading the manuscript. Last but not least, I would like to thank my family (especially Uta, Rainer, Andreas, and Birger Krause, and Ruth and Helmuth Geißler) and my friend Elianne Chatzaki for their encouragement and personal support.

Competing Interests The author has no competing interests to declare that are relevant to the content of this manuscript.

Contents

CHAPTER 1

Introduction

Abstract Dissociation is a multidimensional transdiagnostic phenomenon, generally defined as a disruption of normally integrated mental functions. While the existence of dissociative phenomena is recognized and validated across cultures, a uniform conceptualization of dissociative symptoms and disorders is currently lacking. A common way to classify dissociative experiences is to distinguish between symptoms of detachment (depersonalization, derealization) and compartmentalization. Compartmentalization is a psychological process in which conflicting emotions, thoughts, or memories are mentally separated, which can lead to fragmented emotional experiences, identity disruptions, and memory disturbances. Dissociation may also include dissociative flashbacks (involuntary, unwanted intrusions of sensory, affective, and cognitive information into conscious awareness or behaviour) and dissociative absorption (total immersion in a present activity or event). The severity of dissociative experiences varies considerably, ranging from non-pathological symptoms to dissociative disorders. While some researchers assume that dissociative experiences represent a continuum, others believe there is a clear qualitative distinction between non-clinical dissociation and pathological dissociation. Pathological dissociation is—at least initially—unexpected, unwanted, confusing, and startling. The impact of dissociative symptoms can vary considerably, depending on their severity and the person´s social-psychological, cultural, and psychopathological background.

A. Krause-Utz, *Dissociation in Borderline Personality Disorder*,
https://doi.org/10.1007/978-3-032-06339-7_1

Keywords Definitions · Depersonalization · Derealization · Dissociation · Dissociative absorption

Dissociative experiences can substantially alter the way people feel, think, behave, and perceive the world and themselves. Psychological and somatic functions that are normally coordinated and integrated are temporarily disconnected [1, 2]. These disruptions can manifest in various ways, including profound detachment from oneself and the surrounding (depersonalization, derealization), dissociative absorption, and compartmentalization [3–5]. The severity of dissociative symptoms ranges from normal or milder manifestations in the general population to severe dissociative disorders, such as dissociative identity disorder (DID). Dissociation is not necessarily pathological and can be a self-protective mechanism for dealing with overwhelming situations. It becomes maladaptive and harmful when it critically interferes with daily life, leading to profound distress and significant impairments. Pathological dissociation is not only a feature of dissociative disorders but also occurs in a variety of other mental disorders, including borderline personality disorder (BPD) and post-traumatic stress disorder (PTSD), see [6–13]. Individuals with chronic dissociation usually exhibit characteristics of more than one mental disorder, show more psychosocial impairments and more mental and physical health problems, such as acute or post-traumatic stress symptoms, depression, anxiety, self-harm, and alcohol or substance abuse. The severity of dissociation is associated with more functional impairments and hospital admissions, indicating a higher psychopathological burden [6–13].

In BPD, dissociative symptoms typically occur during acute stress and last from minutes to hours [14, 15]. At the same time, a subgroup of patients with BPD also experience chronic dissociation, such as persistent depersonalization, self-alienation, identity confusion, and memory fragmentations [6]. Since dissociation often occurs in the context of severe emotional dysregulation, psychotic episodes, or self-harm, it may not always receive full attention and might be considered a mere consequence of distress rather than a relevant target symptom in itself. However, there is evidence that acute dissociative symptoms impair emotional and cognitive processes that are relevant to treatment [16–18], see [19]. Higher levels of dissociation predicted poorer response to trauma-focused treatment [20–22] and more future suicide attempts [23], even when controlling for overall symptom severity. Dissociative tendencies in BPD have been associated with altered body representations, pain analgesia [24–28] and reduced threat sensitivity [16, 18], which may contribute to risk-taking behaviours [29, 30]. If not recognized and sufficiently targeted in treatment, persistent dissociation can contribute to more severe manifestations of BPD.

This pivot aims to provide an overview of the current state of knowledge on dissociation in BPD, discussing possible implications for treatment and future research. So far, research explicitly focusing on dissociation in BPD is relatively sparse compared to the extensive literature on dissociative disorders and the dissociative subtype of PTSD. Phenomenological overlaps and the frequent co-occurrence of BPD with PTSD and dissociative disorders can make it difficult to gain a more nuanced understanding of how dissociation affects individuals with a primary BPD diagnosis [8, 10, 31]. Moreover, recent developments towards a dimensional classification of personality disorders have led to changes in the conceptualization of BPD. Rather than considering BPD as a distinct category, dimensional models assume that BPD symptoms occur on a spectrum, with varying degrees of severity [32]. An increasing number of studies is investigating whether dissociative symptoms are part of a complex symptom matrix and how they relate to a broader severity spectrum of BPD features [33–36].

The first part of this pivot introduces relevant definitions and conceptualizations of dissociation. Dissociation is a multifaceted phenomenon that generally refers to disruptions of normally integrated mental functions. While the presence and clinical relevance of dissociative phenomena is recognized across cultures, a uniform classification of dissociative symptoms and disorders is currently lacking. Differences in the conceptualization of dissociation make a clear interpretation of research findings difficult. It is important to highlight that the field is still partly divided, although more and more researchers and clinicians are calling for a transtheoretical perspective of dissociation as a multifaceted phenomenon [37, 38]. Dissociation has been of interest to psychiatry and psychology for more than a century and debates concerning the classification, etiology, and treatment of dissociative disorders are still ongoing. Chronic stress and psychological trauma as well as social-cognitive factors are considered important risk factors for dissociative disorders, which probably develop due to an interplay of various factors [37, 38]. Sleep disturbances, difficulties in recognizing, expressing, and regulating emotions, as well as maladaptive schemas, may be important mechanisms that underlie dissociative tendencies in different disorders. Neurobiological research has offered additional insights into how dissociative states may alter information processing during cognitive tasks and in response to emotionally stressful or threatening material. An overview of these different perspectives and relevant research findings is given. Established screening questionnaires, self-report scales, and clinician-administered structured interviews for dissociative disorders are mentioned, and challenges in the diagnostic process are described. Given the broad spectrum of dissociative experiences, it is important to consider various possible etiological pathways as well as modulating and mediating factors during the assessment of symptoms. Early detection of dissociative symptoms and disorders is important to prevent more serious chronic problems and to offer adequate treatment as early as possible.

The second part of this pivot presents research findings from psychometric, experimental or ecological momentary assessment studies, as well as psychophysical and neuroimaging studies on associations between dissociation and emotion regulation self-referential processing, body perception, and cognitive functioning. There is evidence that chronic dissociative experiences are complexly intertwined with core features of BPD, such as affective instability, unstable self-image, impulsivity, and insecure attachment. These findings underscore the need to understand dissociative symptoms within a larger biosocial framework that considers a complex interplay of developmental trajectories, stressors, and maintaining factors. Ultimately, it emphasizes the need to carefully assess, understand, and treat the diverse manifestations of dissociative symptoms within each individual.

1.1 Dissociation as a Transdiagnostic Multidimensional Construct

Dissociation is a multidimensional construct which encompasses various symptoms. It is generally defined as a disruption of normally integrated functions, such as consciousness, perception, attention, memory, identity, and body representation, which become less amenable to conscious awareness and control [1, 2]. These disruptions can manifest in various ways, both as an acute, temporary state and as a general tendency towards dissociation. In current literature, dissociation is often used as an umbrella term that can refer to both the underlying process and the associated symptoms [39, 40].

The existence of dissociative phenomena is recognized and validated across cultures [41–44]. At the same time, there is no clear consensus on how dissociative symptoms should be conceptualized or classified [1, 15]. Dissociation can have both psychoform and somatoform manifestations [39, 45, 46]. Psychoform dissociation involves disruptions in mental processes, such as consciousness, perception, attention, memory, identity, and emotion. Somatoform dissociation can include medically unexplained neurological or somatic symptoms, such as blindness, aphonia, paralysis, or seizures, which were formally classified as conversion disorders. Currently, the inclusion of conversion symptoms in psychiatric classifications of dissociation is controversial; see Sect. 3.1.3.

1.2 Symptom Domains

The heterogeneity of dissociative symptoms has led to different theoretical perspectives regarding their conceptualization and classification. A common distinction is between symptoms of detachment (depersonalization and derealization) and compartmentalization (separation of mental elements such as emotions, thoughts, or memories) [3]. Other conceptualizations propose a distinction between positive symptoms (intrusions and dissociative flashbacks) and negative symptoms (lack of control and access to normally accessible functions), which may be particularly relevant for pathological forms of dissociation [4, 47, 48].

Spiegel and Cardena [4] proposed three domains of dissociative phenomena. The first category refers to involuntary and unwanted intrusions of sensory, affective, and cognitive information into conscious awareness or behaviour, such as dissociative flashbacks. During dissociative flashbacks, dissociation leads to a loss of continuity in subjective experience. People feel or act as if a past event were happening again, often accompanied by an altered sense of time. In extreme cases, the person completely loses awareness of present surroundings. The second category includes the loss of access to normally amenable information or functions. This refers to a failure to integrate self-referential information and self-attributions and disruptions in autobiographical memories, which can manifest as dissociative amnesia. The third category includes symptoms of depersonalization and derealization, which involve an experiential disconnectedness from oneself (thoughts, feelings, sensations, body, and actions) and/or alienation from the environment. During derealization, people or objects in the surrounding seem unreal, unfamiliar, dreamlike, blurred, lifeless, visually distorted, foggy, or far away. This can include visual perceptions, for example, parts of the own body may appear larger or smaller than usual or not connected to the rest of the body. People with chronic detachment experiences often describe themselves as detached observers, which often involves a deep sense of self-alienation.

Another proposed symptom domain is dissociative absorption or trance, were a person is totally immersed in a present activity or event, while losing connection to reality and the surroundings [5, 49, 50]. Vivid daydreaming, fantasizing, and imaginative involvement are often mentioned as examples of mild non-pathological dissociation [5]. However, severe cases of absorption and maladaptive daydreaming can lead to reduced self-awareness and a disconnection from reality, which can critically interfere with important life domains [49]. This illustrates the broad spectrum of dissociative symptoms and their severity.

1.3 Severity Spectrum

The severity of dissociative experiences ranges considerably, from normal or milder symptoms to pathological expressions of dissociation and dissociative disorders [5, 51, 52]. In general, symptoms should be evaluated in relation to the individual's age, psychological development, and current living situation [47, 53].

Dissociation can be understood as a human process that everyone experiences now and then to some degree, which is not necessarily pathological. Typical examples of normal or milder dissociation include normal daydreaming, getting lost in a book, zoning out in the middle of a conversation, sensory misperceptions when falling asleep, transient gaps in attention and memory when stressed, and the so-called highway hypnosis: switching to autopilot while driving a long highway. Mild symptoms of dissociation do not necessarily cause problems and can help to deal with the complexity of everyday life, such as managing different social role expectations and demands [3, 54, 55]. For highly sensitive individuals dissociation can help to protect themselves from overstimulation. A non-clinical dissociative coping style has been associated with attentional hyperfocus and enhanced working memory capacity [56, 57]. Dissociative absorption overlaps with creative flow experiences, which can lead to exceptional performance and extraordinary achievements [58]. In highly stressful threatening situations when neither fight nor flight is possible, dissociation may be an evolutionary-based survival mechanism and an important prerequisite for necessary developmental adaptations [59–61]; see Sect. 4.1.

Severe forms of dissociation, however, cause significant distress and impairment and critically impact daily life [1, 15, 48, 51]; see Sect. 3. 1. Pathological levels of dissociation are associated with severe mental and physical health problems, maladaptive coping (self-harm, alcohol or substance abuse), suicidal behaviour, more functional impairments and hospital admissions, indicating a high psychopathological burden [6–13]. The majority of studies points to neuropsychological impairments in various domains, including attention, planning, learning and memory; see [19] and Sect. 6.4.

The continuum model states that dissociation exists on a spectrum [1]. If understood as a continuum, gradual transitions from initially mild or adaptive dissociative symptoms to maladaptive pathological processes are possible. Learning-theoretical processes, such as positive and negative reinforcement and generalization can lead to the maintenance of dissociation as a maladaptive coping response [5, 62], see Sect. 5.1.2. The continuum model is useful to understand the broad range of dissociative experiences and the necessity to evaluate both their adaptive and maladaptive functions. Nonetheless, it has been argued that pathological forms of dissociation are not comparable to normative dissociation [5, 51, 55].

The taxonomy by Waller et al. [5] proposes that there is a fundamental difference between non-clinical and pathological dissociation. From this perspective, pathological dissociation is not simply a more severe form of dissociation but qualitatively different from experiences that occur in non-clinical populations. In other words, pathological dissociative experiences go far beyond ordinary dissociative experiences and may involve different underlying mechanisms. One proposed aspect of pathological dissociation is that it is—at least initially—unexpected and unwanted. It represents a startling and intense disruption of normal functioning, which is perceived as fundamentally incompatible with normal functioning [48, 53]. When they first appear, symptoms of dissociation are often scary, alarming, and confusing, which may prevent those affected from sharing their experiences.

There is some evidence that pathological forms of dissociation are associated with different risk factors than less debilitating dissociative symptoms. Research suggests that pathological dissociation is more strongly related to psychological trauma, especially emotional, physical, and sexual abuse and neglect in childhood [45]. However, a direct comparisons of findings is difficult because different forms of dissociation may not be adequately captured by established standardized scales [37, 63]. Moreover, the development of dissociative disorders typically involves an interplay of many factors, including genetic neurobiological vulnerabilities; see Sect. 4.

CHAPTER 2

Mental Disorders Associated with Dissociation

Abstract Dissociative disorders are mental disorders in which dissociation is the central feature that causes significant distress and/or impairments in important areas of life. Both the Diagnostic and Statistical Manual of Mental Disorders (DSM-5) and the International Classification of Diseases (ICD-11) recognize depersonalization derealization disorder, dissociative amnesia with or without diagnostic fugue, and dissociative identity disorder as dissociative disorders and provide additional categories for unspecified or other specified dissociative disorders. The ICD-11 includes a dissociative neurological symptom disorder for medically unexplained neurological symptoms that were formally classified as conversion symptoms. The DSM-5 renamed conversion disorder to functional neurological symptom disorder which is placed in the separate category of somatic symptom disorders. It is increasingly recognized that pathological dissociation occurs not only in dissociative disorders but also in a variety of other mental disorders, including borderline personality disorder (BPD) and post-traumatic stress disorder (PTSD). Phenomenological overlap and frequent co-occurrence of these disorders with dissociative disorders can complicate the diagnostic and therapeutic process.

Keywords Borderline personality disorder · Dissociative disorders · International classification of diseases · Post-traumatic stress disorder · Statistical manual of mental disorders

A. Krause-Utz, *Dissociation in Borderline Personality Disorder*,
https://doi.org/10.1007/978-3-032-06339-7_2

Dissociative disorders are characterized by high levels of recurrent dissociation that critically interfere with psychosocial functioning in daily life [1, 15]. While individuals with dissociative disorders report the highest level of dissociation, clinically relevant dissociative symptoms also occur in a variety of other mental disorders, including PTSD and BPD [6, 11]. According to a comprehensive meta-analysis of 216 studies with 15,219 participants from nineteen different diagnostic groups, patients with dissociative disorders, particularly DID, report the highest levels of dissociation, followed by PTSD, BPD, conversion disorder, somatic symptom disorder, substance-related and addictive disorders, eating disorders, schizophrenia, obsessive–compulsive disorders, depressive disorders, anxiety disorders, and bipolar disorder [6]. Findings from this meta-analysis highlight the transdiagnostic nature of dissociation. The fifth edition of the Diagnostic and Statistical Manual of Mental Disorders (DSM-5) has introduced a dissociative subtype of PTSD to acknowledge the relevance of persistent dissociation, particularly depersonalization and derealization, in subgroups of patients with PTSD. Sar [15] proposed the inclusion of a dissociative subtype for depression, based on clinical observations and empirical findings that dissociation often co-occurs with chronic and treatment-resistant forms of depression, particularly in individuals with severe childhood trauma [64–66]. Dissociation might also occur in neurodevelopmental disorders, including autism spectrum disorders (ASD) and attention deficit hyperactivity disorders (ADHD), although more research in this field is needed [67, 68]. Traits like alexithymia (difficulty identifying and describing emotional states), challenges with interoception (awareness of bodily sensations), and protective shutdowns can occur both in ASD and chronic dissociative disorders [67]. Attention deficits, mind wandering, hyper-focus and executive dysfunction in ADHD may be reminiscent of dissociative phenomena [68], although they appear to have different neurobiological bases [17, 69, 70].

All in all, it is increasingly recognized that dissociation is a transdiagnostic phenomenon that occurs in various mental disorders, not only dissociative disorders. Individuals who experience chronic dissociation often show signs of more than one dissociative disorder, symptoms of PTSD, (borderline) personality disorders, anxiety and mood disorders, eating disorders, substance use disorders, and sleep disorders, and there can be diagnostic shifts over time.

The following sections provide an overview of the currently recognized dissociative disorders in International Classification of Diseases (ICD-11) and DSM-5, the dissociative subtype of PTSD, complex PTSD, and some proposed additions. Dissociation is highly common in BPD, but it is only one of many symptoms and neither a necessary nor defining one. To account for the wide variety of BPD symptoms, a general overview of the disorder is provided in Sect. 1.1.2. Afterwards, challenges of differential diagnosis are discussed.

2.1 Dissociative Disorders

Dissociative disorders are mental disorders in which dissociation is the central feature that causes significant distress and/or impairments in one or more important life domains. Currently, both the DSM-5 [1] and the ICD-11 [15] recognize depersonalization derealization disorder, dissociative amnesia with or without diagnostic fugue, and DID as dissociative disorders, and offer additional categories for other specified or unspecified dissociative disorders. The ICD-11 further includes a dissociative neurological symptom disorder diagnosis [15]. Symptoms that were classified as hysteria in the late nineteenth and much of the twentieth centuries [54, 71, 72] and listed as conversion disorder in earlier versions of psychiatric classification systems [14, 15] are included here. In contrast, the DSM-5 categorizes these symptoms under functional neurological symptom disorder, placed within the somatic symptom disorders category. This emphasizes the possibility that there is an unknown medical explanation for neurological-like symptoms without identifiable neurological damage and that the maladaptive reactions to the symptoms is at the core of the disorder [1]. Both the ICD-11 and DSM-5 acknowledge that symptoms are real even though they are not necessarily explained by a known neurological disease and that they cause significant distress.

2.1.1 Epidemiology

The estimated prevalence of dissociative disorders is between 1 and 4% in the general population [64, 73–75]. Transient episodes of depersonalization and derealization (for example, due to physical and emotional exhaustion, physical illness, or a substance that makes people feel tired, detached, or drowsy) are much more common than depersonalization derealization disorder [1, 64]. Nonetheless, numerous independent studies from different countries have clearly demonstrated that pathological dissociation constitutes a common mental health problem not only in clinical practice but also in the community, see [64]. In clinical settings, prevalences of dissociative disorders are usually higher, with approximately 10% of psychiatric patients meeting the diagnostic criteria [64, 76, 77]. In emergency departments and inpatient treatment units prevalences are usually higher; one study found up to 35% of patients with a primary diagnosis of depression, somatization disorder, and BPD had a co-occurring dissociative disorder [78]. Data derived from epidemiological studies also support a relationship between adverse childhood experiences and dissociative disorders [64].

Worldwide, dissociative disorders are more frequently diagnosed in women than in men although empirical studies suggest that dissociative symptoms occur equally in both biological sexes [79]. Men were found to enter the health system less often and may be less likely to report symptoms or ask for help for these problems. A growing number of studies has shown that dissociative symptoms are found in different cultures [43, 44, 80], including non-Western countries and regions, such as Taiwan and Hong Kong [34, 81–85].

Prevalence estimates were found to vary depending on the diagnostic tool and criteria used. As discussed in Sect. 3.3, this includes the risk of both underdiagnosis, misdiagnosis, and overdiagnosis. Underdiagnosis is believed to be more common, especially for DID [64, 86]. Since general psychiatric assessments do not cover criteria for dissociative disorders, previous large-scale epidemiological studies might have led to biased results and an underestimation of prevalences [64]. Sar [64] discusses that the relatively high number of co-occurring diagnoses in patients with chronic dissociation and symptom overlap with PTSD and BPD may prevent clinicians from recognizing the dissociative disorder in the overall picture [64].

2.1.2 *Cultural Differences*

There is evidence for sociocultural differences in the manifestation and interpretation of dissociative symptoms, as well as the choice of diagnostic instrument, which can lead to differences in prevalence estimates [75]. The manifestation and presentation of dissociative symptoms can be influenced by the individual's cultural background. Symptoms that are regarded as normal in one cultural context are interpreted as unusual in another [15, 87, 88]. In some spiritual or meditative practices, intentionally induced dissociative states are a desired outcome. According to the ICD-11, (possession) trance disorder shows considerable cross-cultural variation regarding the presence of dissociative sensory and motor alterations and behaviours during the altered state [15]. Concerning DID, prolonged intercultural contact may shape the characteristics of dissociative identities with respect to spoken language and clothing style. In some societies, the tendency towards dissociative responses to stress may be increased due to less individualistic conceptions of the self.

2.1.3 Diagnostic Criteria

General diagnostic criteria for dissociative disorders are the presence of recurrent dissociative symptoms that are not primarily caused by a substance, drug, or medication (e.g., blackouts and chaotic behaviour during substance intoxication), and not due to a somatic condition (e.g., temporary global amnesia or traumatic brain injury). Another general diagnostic criterion is that symptoms are not better explained by another disorder in which dissociative symptoms can occurs, such as acute stress disorder, PTSD, panic disorder, depressive disorder, somatic symptom disorder, schizophrenia, or neurocognitive disorder. As discussed in Sect. 1.6, differential diagnosis can be challenging.

Depersonalization derealization disorder (DPDR) is characterized by recurrent or persistent episodes of detachment (depersonalization and/or derealization), which critically interfere with social, occupational, or other domains of functioning [1]. These recurrent experiences feel extremely distressing and can be accompanied by anxiety, depression, and time distortions. Individuals may feel like an outside observer of their own life, emotionally numb, and disconnected from the own body, actions, and speech, as if out of control. Derealization may involve distorted perceptions of surroundings (as blurry, distorted, dreamlike, or unusually clear), and chronic feelings of isolation, as if separated by a glass wall. Prevalence rates for DPDR range between 1 and 2% in the general population and 5% in clinical populations [64, 73].

Dissociative amnesia (DA) is the inability to remember important autobiographical information, mostly involving past events (retrograde amnesia) that are related to a highly stressful or traumatic situation [1]. The amnesia can occur gradually or abruptly, last for minutes or hours or even for years. It can be either localized (selective amnesia for specific events) or generalized (amnesia for an entire part of life history). Symptoms can be accompanied by dissociative fugue, unexpected traveling without clear purpose, confusion, and the establishment of a new identity at a different place. Prevalences range for dissociative amnesia and fugue range from 0.2 to 7.3% but are not well-established [see 46].

Dissociative identity disorder is often mentioned as the most severe and chronic form of pathological dissociation, as it involves a clear and pervasive fragmentation of identity into at least two relatively enduring distinct personality states that evidently influence a person´s behaviour is present. This fragmentation is associated with a pervasive discontinuity in perception, cognition, self-control, and sensorimotor functioning, and accompanied by memory gaps that cannot be explained by ordinary forgetfulness. The fragmentation of identity can lead to clear changes in behaviour, such as sudden fluctuations in skills, knowledge, hobbies, and styles, or handwriting. Memory gaps can concern both personal autobiographical information and everyday events.

The presentation of symptoms can be highly diverse. The ICD-11 gives the option for diagnosing partial DID if symptom presentations include non-dominant personality states which do not recurrently take executive control of the individual's consciousness and functioning [15]. In the DSM, these partial forms may be diagnosed as "other specified dissociative disorder" (OSDD) [1]. Estimated prevalences of DID vary, with approximately 1–1.5% of the general population and 1–7.5% of the clinical population meeting the criteria [64, 90, 91].

The ICD-11 further lists dissociative trance and possession trance disorder as dissociative disorders, characterised by an acute narrowing or complete loss of awareness of immediate surroundings, typically accompanied by stereotypical movements, transient paralysis, or unconsciousness. The acute constriction or complete loss of awareness typically manifests as a very severe lack of responsiveness or insensitivity to environmental stimuli. The person may feel that their personal identity is being replaced by an external identity, which is unwanted and causes significant distress or dysfunction. These states of altered consciousness and personal identity are not part of a generally accepted cultural or religious practice. Conditions, such as delirium and epilepsy must be ruled out as well. The separation between trance disorder and possession disorder in the ICD-11 reflects the distinctive feature in possession trance disorder wherein the usual sense of personal identity is replaced by an external identity attributed to the influence of a spirit, power, deity or other spiritual entity.

Compared to trance disorder, possession trance disorder involves a greater range of more complex behaviours. Prevalences are not well-established and controversial, particularly due to cultural and theoretical differences in how these phenomena are understood and classified [87].

The ICD-11 also includes a category of dissociative neurological symptom disorders. This category consists of twelve subtypes concerning the predominant cognitive, sensory, or motor symptoms that imply an involuntary discontinuity in the normal integration of these functions and are not consistent with another recognized mental disorder, disease of the nervous system, or medical condition [15]. Symptoms do not occur exclusively in the context of another dissociative disorder and are not due to the effects of a substance or medication on the central nervous system, or a Sleep–Wake disorder. Somatoform dissociation is therefore still recognized in the ICD-11, but references to the term "conversion" are removed.

In the DSM-5, conversion disorder is renamed "functional neurological symptom disorder", with the intent to emphasize the incompatibility between symptoms and currently known neurological conditions [1]. This is aimed at providing a more nuanced understanding of these conditions, moving away from a solely psychological explanation and focusing on the neurological symptoms and their impact on the individual's functioning. For the diagnosis of functional neurologic disorder (formally conversion disorder) in DSM-5 it is not required anymore that there is a temporal link between the onset of symptoms and a psychological factor or stressors. Symptoms may include weakness and/or paralysis, non-epileptic seizures, speech or visual impairment, swallowing difficulty, sensory disturbances, movement disorders, and cognitive symptoms. Criteria are the presence of one or more neurologic symptoms (either motor or sensory) that are incompatible with currently recognized neurological or medical conditions and that are not better explained by another medical or mental disorder. Symptoms causes clinically significant distress or impairment in social, occupational, or other important areas of functioning or warrants medical evaluation. The disorder now belongs to the category of "somatic symptom and related disorders", formerly known as "somatoform disorders" [1].

In the category of dissociative disorders, the DSM-5 has two more diagnostic subcategories, which replaced the category of Dissociative Disorder Not Otherwise Specified (DDNOS) in former versions of the

DSM: "other specified dissociative disorders" (OSDD) and "unspecified dissociative disorders" [1]. Symptoms of DID or other dissociative phenomena that do not fully meet the criteria for a specific dissociative disorder can be classified here. Further examples include chronic and recurrent syndromes of mixed dissociative symptoms, identity disturbance due to prolonged and intense coercive persuasion (for example, brainwashing, indoctrination in captivity or under torture, long-term political imprisonment, or terror organizations), trance, and acute dissociative reactions to stressful events that typically last less than 1 month. In the DSM category OSDD, the clinician can further specify why a clinical picture does not meet the criteria for a specific dissociative disorder and how dissociative symptoms cause clinically significant distress or impairment in important life areas. The ICD-11 also includes a category of "other specified dissociative disorders" [15]. The OSDD category is the most frequently used way to diagnose dissociative disorders in DSM, being used in 30–65% of cases [64]. This relatively high prevalence in clinical and community settings has been interpreted as a sign that more diagnostic categories as well as broader definitions of identity disruptions in DID are needed [64].

2.2 The Dissociative Subtype of Post-traumatic Stress Disorder

A dissociative subtype of PTSD was introduced in the DSM-5 for patients who repeatedly experience depersonalization and derealization. Post-traumatic stress disorder develops in approximately 5.6% of individuals exposed to a traumatic event or a series of events [92]. Traumatic experiences are highly common and it is natural that people experience a wide range of acute stress reactions after experiencing a potentially traumatizing event (PTE); these symptoms usually subside after a certain time [93]. In those who develop PTSD, symptoms persist for more than a month after the traumatic event. Core symptoms of PTSD include re-experiencing (recurrent involuntary intrusions of the traumatic events or flashback memories), avoidance of trauma-related information, negative mood and cognitions, and hyperarousal. Individuals with the dissociative subtype of PTSD have recurrent symptoms of depersonalization and derealization in addition to other PTSD symptoms. Only symptoms of derealization and depersonalization distinguished this group from PTSD patients without the dissociative subtype, while individuals with PTSD generally experience a wide range of dissociative symptoms [94]. According to a systematic review from 2017, prevalence rates for the dissociative subtype ranged from 6 (veteran samples) to 44.6% (survivors of sexual abuse by family members), with a mean prevalence of 20.26% [95]. Systematic reviews suggest that male biological sex, higher age, racial background, prior traumatic exposure (especially childhood sexual and physical abuse) [95], symptom severity, comorbidity, suicidality, as well as multiple exposure to different types of trauma [94] are associated with the dissociative subtype in some—albeit not all—of the included studies.

2.3 Complex Post-traumatic Stress Disorder in ICD-11

The ICD-11 does not include a dissociative subtype of PTSD. Unlike the DSM-5, it includes the diagnosis of complex post-traumatic stress disorder (CPTSD) [15], which has been linked to high levels of dissociation [96–100]. In ICD-11, CPTSD and PTSD exist as "sibling diagnoses" that both require the presence of PTSD symptoms—traumatic re-experiencing, avoidance of traumatic reminders, and hyperarousal (sense of threat). In addition to these symptoms, CPTSD includes so-called disturbances of self-organization (DSO) in three domains: emotional numbing and dysregulation, profound negative self-perceptions as guilty or worthless, and avoidance of intimate relationships or emotional detachment in relationships. Persistent dissociative symptoms were included in the initial formulation of CPTSD by Judith Herman [101]. Due to a lack of consistent empirical evidence, dissociation was not included in the ICD-11 CPTSD diagnosis in 2018 [102]. Since then, researchers have continued to examine the presence of dissociation in CPTSD. Several studies found significantly higher levels of dissociative experiences in patients with CPTSD than in those with "classic" PTSD and in traumatized individuals who did not develop a mental disorder [96–100]. A study by Jowett et al. [100] suggests that dissociation is positively linked to CPTSD symptom severity in individuals who experienced childhood trauma. Hyland et al. [99] investigated whether ICD-11 CPTSD symptoms exist independently of dissociation in a nationally representative sample of adults ($N = 1020$). Using latent class analysis, they found that ICD-11 CPTSD symptoms can occur without corresponding dissociative experiences. However, when CPTSD symptoms and dissociative experiences occurred together, this was associated with poorer mental health outcomes and higher levels of functional impairment. Similarly, Fung et al. [43] found that dissociative symptoms were found in 42.3% of 165 intervention seeking individuals with CPTSD and uniquely associated with depressive symptoms and work and social impairments. These findings suggest that CPTSD is not a dissociative disorder, but it is important to recognize dissociation in people with CPTSD, because it appears to indicate more functional impairments [98].

Unlike the DSM-5, the ICD-11 does not have a strict "A criterion" (also known as "trauma criterion") for the cause of PTSD symptoms. The DSM-5 requires that PTSD symptom develop after exposure to actual or threatened death, serious injury, or sexual violence in a direct and/or indirect way by witnessing in person or learning that it occurred to others [1]. This means that psychologically threatening events, such as bullying or stalking, do not meet this criterion unless there is serious physical injury, threatened bodily harm, or threatened death. In its 'expanded' trauma definition, the ICD-11 recognizes the potential impact of psychologically threatening events, including emotional abuse, rejection, and neglect, on the development of PTSD [103]. The diagnosis of PTSD can be made if symptoms are related to a past event or series of events, which was/were "extremely threatening or horrific", including events which do not unambiguously pose direct or indirect threat to life and physical safety [15]. Research by Hyland et al. [103] suggests that the ICD-11 approach of providing clinical guidance rather than a formal definition of trauma has not led to an inflated prevalence of PTSD in a nationally representative sample from Ireland ($N = 1020$) [103]. Prevalence estimates for CPTSD range from 0.5 to 7.7% in the general population but are higher (around 36%) in clinical samples [93]; see [31].

2.4 Proposed Additions

2.4.1 Developmental Trauma Disorder

The proposal for Developmental Trauma Disorder (DTD) for children and adolescents, who are repeatedly exposed to developmentally adverse interpersonal trauma, was made [104]. While this proposal was not adopted in the DSM, it played an important role in the establishment of the CPTSD diagnosis in the ICD-11, see [105]. An updated model proposes four symptom clusters: severe emotional or somatic dysregulation (extreme distress and impaired recovery from distress), attentional or behavioural dysregulation (impaired ability to initiate or sustain goal-directed behaviour and consistent problems in independently starting and completing actions designed to achieve personal goals), extreme risk-taking or reckless or careless behaviour, and impulsive aggression [106–108]. Dissociation is a proposed core feature of DTD, which is included in the domain of affective and somatic dysregulation. Within this framework, it is assumed that dissociation develops within a complex psychological, biological, and relational adaptation to early childhood trauma and disorganized attachment experiences with primary caregivers, see also Sect. 4.1.3.2. Traumatic experiences during sensitive phases of psychosocial development can lead to a profound pattern of emotional and cognitive-behavioural dysregulation [106–108].

2.4.2 Dissociative Subtype of Depression

A dissociative subtype of depression was proposed, based on clinical observations and empirical findings that dissociation often co-occurs with chronic and treatment-resistant forms of depression, particularly in individuals with severe childhood trauma [64–66]. This subtype has not been officially recognized in psychiatric classification systems and diagnostic manuals. Phenomenologically, dissociative depression has been described as a highly chronic but irregular depressive mood with an early onset, which does not entirely fit diagnostic criteria for dysthymia or clear-cut recurrent depressive episodes and is less responsive to standard treatments [65, 66]. Findings suggest that dissociation is more common in individuals with chronic depression after childhood trauma. More research is needed to disentangle the effects of early trauma and co-occurring conditions, such as BPD [65, 66].

2.4.3 Maladaptive Daydreaming as a Dissociative Disorder

Maladaptive daydreaming is a frequently under-recognized aspect of complex dissociative disorders [109–111]. Based on growing research in the field, it has recently been proposed that maladaptive daydreaming should be included as a dissociative disorder in psychiatric manuals [111]. Maladaptive daydreaming is characterized by excessive, vivid, and immersive daydreaming that negatively impacts daily life. Normal daydreaming can be a temporary relief from aversive feelings, while maladaptive daydreaming is excessive, compulsive, and highly detrimental to one's life.

Individuals with maladaptive daydreaming may find it hard concentrate on daily demands and prioritize daydreaming over other responsibilities and social connections. In contrast to normal daydreaming, maladaptive daydreaming involves excessive fantasizing and immersion in mental imagery of alternative realities, often through repetitive stereotypical behaviours, which distracts from problem-solving and self-care, involves significant distress, and leads to significant impairments in important areas of life. In this respect, maladaptive daydreaming fits the criteria for dissociative disorders in psychiatric manuals [111].

2.5 Borderline Personality Disorder

Borderline personality disorder (BPD) is characterized by marked instability of emotions, self-image, and relationships [1]. Dissociation is a common symptom of BPD, but it is not experienced by every person with the disorder, similar to other symptoms such as self-harm or aggressive outbursts. The diagnosis can be based on a variety of symptoms that generally relate to three core domains: emotion dysregulation, unstable identity, and interpersonal disturbances [112]. Emotion dysregulation involves heightened emotional sensitivity, intense, highly unstable, and long-lasting emotions, and the use of maladaptive emotional coping strategies, such as self-harm. Identity disturbances include a markedly unstable sense of self and a lack of consistent personal goals or values. Interpersonal problems often arise from a hypervigilance to social clues signaling potential threat and rejection and involve pervasive distrust, feelings of loneliness, alienation and social exclusion. Behavioural manifestations, such as repetitive non-suicidal self-injury, suicidal behaviours, and anger outbursts, should be understood as maladaptive coping attempts to deal with these underlying problems [112, 113]. Dissociative symptoms often co-occur with other BPD symptoms, such as emotional dysregulation, identity disturbance, and self-harm [10, 33]. It is currently assumed that BPD develops from an interplay of genetic, neurobiological vulnerability and environmental stressors, including both trauma-related and non-trauma related pathways [112]. Dissociation should be understood in this biosocial framework.

2.5.1 Epidemiology and Course of Symptoms

Prevalences of BPD range between 0.7 and 2.7% in community settings; 2–3% of adolescents (12–17 years) and 0–4% of adults above the age of forty meet criteria for the diagnosis [114, 115]. Prevalences are substantially higher in inpatient settings (22.4%) and in outpatient settings (11.8%). While more women than men are diagnosed with BPD in clinical settings, there are mixed findings regarding sex or gender differences in the general population. Similar to dissociative disorders, men are less likely to seek medical help and may be less likely to report symptoms of BPD [112]. Common comorbidities include PTSD (30–70%), anxiety disorders (84.5%) mood disorders [82.7%; bipolar disorder I: 21.6%, bipolar II: 37.7%)], and substance use disorders (78.2%) [116–120] as well as dissociative disorders (30–72%), see Sect. 1.5.3.

First symptoms typically occur in adolescence or early adulthood, around the age of thirteen [112] and often co-occur with symptoms of internalizing disorders (depression and anxiety) and externalizing disorders (conduct problems, hyperactivity, and substance use), even when psychiatric comorbidities are accounted for [121]. Identifying early signs of BPD and treating them at an early stage can reduce the progression of functional impairments [122, 123]. For decades, BPD was considered untreatable, but advances in its understanding and management have led to earlier detection and better treatment outcomes [112]. In a recent meta-analytic review of naturalistic and post-treatment follow-up studies in adults, a mean diagnostic remission rate of 60% (95% IC: 49–71%) was found, suggesting that considerable psychosocial functional improvement can be achieved with treatment [124]. Younger age at baseline was associated with higher remission rates at follow-up, which highlights the importance of early diagnosis and intervention. Long-term functional outcomes appear to be worse in women, possibly due to the effects of abuse histories and gender roles [124]. Predictors of recovery include stable functioning as a parent, spouse or partner [125]. Outcomes vary significantly among individuals—a subgroup of patients appears to suffer more persistent psychosocial impairments over time [86] and this may also be linked to dissociation; see Sect. 1.5.3. There is a high degree of fluidity with changes between remission and recurrences of symptoms [126]. Many patients, who achieve symptomatic remission still suffer from long-term problems with social integration and experience chronic feelings of emptiness and loneliness, fear of abandonment, and intolerance to aloneness [112]. Only small improvements in social functioning can be seen after otherwise successful psychotherapeutic interventions [127, 128]. Family members of individuals with BPD also often report a high burden associated with grief and helplessness [129] and may profit from family interventions [130, 131].

2.5.2 *Diagnostic Criteria*

In the last decade, there have been substantial changes in the classification of personality disorders [32]. Currently, three different classification systems are available for diagnosing BPD in adolescents and adults. The DSM-5 continues to offer the traditional categorical system, which requires at least five of the following nine polythetic criteria for the BPD diagnosis to be met: (1) fear of abandonment, (2) unstable relationships, (3) unstable self-image, (4) potentially self-damaging impulsivity, (5) recurrent suicidal behaviour and threats or acts of self-harm, (6) affective instability, (7) chronic feelings of emptiness, (8) inappropriate anger including impulsive aggression, and (9) transient dissociative states and/or paranoid ideation. The DSM-5 offers this categorical model with the traditional criteria in Section II, next to an Alternative Model of Personality Disorders (AMPD) in Section III. The AMPD involves a stepwise diagnostic process. First, the general level of personality function (identity and interpersonal functioning) is determined. Secondly, the presence of five personality trait domains (negative affectivity, detachment, psychoticism, antagonism, and disinhibition) can be described; see [132, 133]. A BPD diagnosis can be determined when the client shows high levels of negative affectivity (emotional lability, anxiousness, separation insecurity, depression), antagonism (hostility), and disinhibition (impulsivity and risk-taking; at least one symptom must be impulsivity, risk-taking, or hostility). Dissociative symptoms most likely refer to the domain of psychoticism [134]; see Sect. 1.5.3.

The ICD-11 uses an entirely dimensional conceptualization of personality disorders in general and BPD in specific. It moved away from the categorical approach and conceptualizes personality disorders as extreme variations of common personality traits. Similar to the AMPD in DSM-5, the clinician first determines the general personality dysfunction (no impairment, personality difficulty, mild, moderate, and severe). Five trait domain qualifiers (negative affectivity, detachment, disinhibition, dissociability, anakastia) can be used to describe the way personality functioning is impaired. A "borderline pattern" can be used to describe the symptom pattern that aligns with the former BPD diagnosis, including the presence of stress-related dissociative symptoms. In addition, the following symptoms are associated with BPD: a negative self-view (as inadequate, guilty, bad, contemptible), a deep sense of loneliness and alienation, distrust, misinterpretation of social signals, and increased rejection sensitivity [32]. It is recommended that symptom assessment and psychoeducation should be initiated as soon as possible during an open, transparent, and collaborative diagnostic process [135].

2.5.3 Dissociation in BPD

Dissociation is experienced by approximately 75–80% of people with BPD [7, 9]. According to the DSM-5 and ICD-11, dissociative symptoms typically occur during states of acute stress [1] or in situations of high affective arousal [15] and last between minutes and hours in BPD. A subgroup of patients with BPD also experiences persistent dissociation, including chronic symptoms of detachment (depersonalization, derealization) and compartmentalization (memory and identity fragmentations) [6]. Dissociation severity is associated with more functional impairments, more hospital admissions [136], a higher number of co-occurring mental and physical health problems or comorbidities, especially post-traumatic stress and psychotic symptoms, and more overall distress [81]. Moreover, dissociation appears to be more prevalent and more persistent in BPD patients with trauma histories [136], including sexual abuse and rape in childhood and adulthood [137], which might be due to higher comorbidity with PTSD and complex PTSD in this group.

Approximately 30–72% of patients with BPD meet diagnostic criteria for a comorbid dissociative disorder; see [9, 64, 138]. Estimated prevalences vary depending on the study population and diagnostic tools, but appear to be higher in patients with severe trauma, as well as in inpatient treatment units and psychiatric emergency ward assessments. Research suggests that individuals who meet criteria for both BPD and DID present with more severe dissociative symptoms, more psychopathological symptoms (including difficulties in emotion regulation, self-harm, substance abuse, and suicidal behaviour), and more trauma histories than individuals who were diagnosed with either diagnosis alone [139].

Dissociative experiences often co-occur with psychotic symptoms in BPD [81]. A latent class analysis of 504 patients with a BPD diagnosis based on the categorical model found three symptom classes or latent subgroups [140]. A small "non-labile" group showed low levels of dissociative symptoms and low affective instability. The second (larger) group was characterized by high levels of dissociative and paranoid symptoms, low abandonment fears and identity disturbance. The third group was characterized by high efforts to avoid abandonment and interpersonal aggression.

A recent study investigated the relationship between the maladaptive personality facets of the DSM-5 Alternative Model of Personality Disorder and recurrent dissociative experiences (depersonalization, derealization, dissociative amnesia, and absorption) in a sample of 178 patients with BPD based on the DSM-IV diagnosis [134]. Findings suggest that patients with frequent dissociative experiences show higher levels in the domain of psychoticism (unusual behaviours and beliefs and perceptual dysregulation), more withdrawal, lower levels of impulsivity and irritability, lower levels of callousness and low levels of avoidance. This suggests that dissociative symptoms should be understood within the domain of psychoticism as specifier. All in all, these findings highlight the need to further improve the understanding and treatment of dissociation in subgroups of BPD patients.

2.6 Phenomenological Overlap and Differential Diagnosis

The phenomenological overlaps and frequent co-occurrence of BPD with trauma-related and dissociative disorders can complicate the diagnostic process; see [31]. Emotional dysregulation, negative self-image, identity disturbances, and self-destructive behaviours occur in all these disorders and may be shared transdiagnostic features that have also been associated with persistent dissociation, especially in groups with complex symptom presentations and trauma histories, see [8, 10, 31, 64]. Adverse childhood experiences, such as abuse and neglect by primary caregivers, and interpersonal victimization in adolescence and adulthood may be a shared etiological pathway. At the same time, BPD and dissociative disorders are currently not classified as trauma-related disorders and not necessarily caused by traumatic stress [141]. Several researchers have proposed features that could help distinguish between dissociative disorders, PTSD, and BPD as well as psychotic disorders.

2.6.1 Borderline Personality Disorder and DID

There is substantial overlap between BPD and DID with regard to identity disturbances, emotional dysregulation, self-harm, and dissociation, see [8, 10, 31, 64]. It is commonly empathized that identity fragmentations in BPD are less stable and also less obvious in clinical assessment than in DID [8]. While it has been shown that severe identity disturbances in BPD include a highly fragmented, poorly integrated and polarized sense of self with distorted body and self-perception, symptoms of dissociative compartmentalization are typically more pervasive in DID. It has been pointed out that individuals with BPD tend to have a fluctuating sense of self, while DID involves more stable and distinct identity states [8, 13]. Korzekwa and Dell [13] emphasize that dissociative states in BPD typically resemble episodic mental and physical breakdowns, while DID involves a more stable and consistent compartmentalization of experiences and more active mental efforts to block emotions. Sar [65] further argued that DID involves more memory fragmentations. Memory gaps, including distinct amnesic barriers between identity states, are seen as a hallmark of DID but not BPD.

With respect to emotional dysregulation, both BPD and DID are characterized by difficulties managing intense emotions. Brand and Lanius [8] argue that BPD includes more rapid mood swings, heightened sensitivity and reactivity to interpersonal stressors, highly unstable emotions, difficulty soothing oneself, and impulsive self-harming emotional coping attempts. Nonetheless, Brand and Lanius [8] view BPD as a disorder of "emotional under-regulation". In contrast, individuals with DID usually show symptoms of "emotional over-regulation", associated with a reduced ability to express emotions or body states. However, not all individuals with BPD exhibit markedly dysregulated behaviour [142]. Some people with the disorder show highly inhibited, constrained, or rigid ("over-controlled") behaviour [143], and this "hidden" or "quiet" variant of BPD is often overlooked [112]. Moreover, in BPD, states of emotional under-regulation may alternate with states of emotional over-regulation, chronic states of emptiness, and numbing and it is not clear how this is related to dissociation [144].

2.6.2 *Borderline Personality Disorder, PTSD, and CPTSD*

Borderline personality disorders, PTSD, and CPTSD share similarly large phenomenological overlaps, and the disorders can be difficult to distinguish at the symptom level, especially when there is a history of cumulative interpersonal trauma [145]; see [31]. Unlike BPD, PTSD, and CPTSD are trauma-related disorders that are clearly attributable to traumatic experiences. At the same time, rates of interpersonal trauma in BPD are very high [146]. Several studies used latent class analysis or latent profile analysis to show that BPD, PTSD, and CPTSD have distinguishing features and are distinct syndromes [147–149]. Reviewing the existing literature to date, Ford and Courtois [31] concluded that BPD, PTSD, and CPTSD are distinct mental health conditions but often co-occur. When occurring in isolation, BPD is associated with more instability in emotions, self-image, and behaviours (more impulsive and unstable relationships alternating between enmeshment and disengagement, more fear of abandonment), while CPTSD involves more intimacy avoidance and detachment in relationships. Based on their literature review, Ford and Courtois [31] propose that PTSD, CPTSD, and BPD may represent a continuum, with increasing psychopathological severity from PTSD to CPTSD and BPD. Since this hypothesis has not yet been directly tested, further research is needed. As an alternative hypothesis, Ford and Courtois [31] propose that BPD may develop as an independent mental health condition that sensitizes a person to a greater impact of trauma exposure, increasing the risk for PTSD or CPTSD.

Ford and Courtois [31] further discuss that some clinicians and individuals with lived experience view the CPTSD diagnosis as less stigmatizing than BPD due to misperceptions and negative stereotypes associated with the latter. While attitudes towards BPD have changed to a more positive empathic understanding of the disorder, the diagnosis still faces considerable stigma, whereas CPTSD may elicit more sympathy and compassion, being the consequence of prolonged or repeated trauma. However, avoiding BPD diagnosis can perpetuate stigma. When communicated openly, with knowledge, empathy, compassion, and professional understanding, the BPD diagnosis can be a relief and help initiate adequate treatment [112, 135].

2.6.3 *Dissociation and Psychosis*

Dissociation is associated with psychotic experiences, particularly hallucinations [150–154]. Psychosis involves altered perceptions that are similar to dissociative experiences but it is characterized by a full loss of contact with reality or a misinterpretation of reality [1, 15]. While dissociation and psychosis are distinct mental health conditions, they can co-occur, and their differentiation is an important part of the diagnostic process in clinical and forensic settings.

A meta-analysis of 58 non-clinical studies (16,557 participants) and 46 clinical studies (3879 patients) revealed a robust association between dissociation and positive psychotic symptoms (hallucinations, delusions, paranoid ideation, and disorganization), with a larger effect in non-clinical samples [154]. Symptom-specific associations with negative symptoms were small or not significant. These findings show that dissociative phenomena are not only robustly related to hallucinations but also to other positive symptoms and suggest that certain psychotic symptoms might even be better conceptualized as dissociative in nature. At the same time, addressing dissociative symptoms might also be beneficial for managing psychosis.

In dissociative disorders, PTSD, and BPD, psychotic symptoms, particularly auditory hallucinations (hearing voices), visual hallucinations, and paranoid delusions, often occur together with dissociative symptoms, but also in isolation [152–155]. Unlike in schizophrenia-spectrum disorders, reality testing is usually intact in dissociative, trauma-related disorders, and BPD [150]. However, Tschoeke et al. [150] emphasize that psychotic symptoms in BPD and trauma-related disorders are comparable to positive symptoms in schizophrenia-spectrum disorders, posing a profound challenge for differential diagnosis in clinical and forensic settings.

Auditory hallucinations can manifest in various ways, as a single voice or multiple voices that comment, communicate instructions, comfort, or offend. Voice hearing is not uncommon in healthy samples and some researchers believe that it represents a continuum from non-clinical to clinical manifestations. However, voice hearing in dissociative disorders, particularly DID, usually exhibits higher complexity and autonomy [155]. Brand and Lanius [8] argue that auditory-verbal hallucinations in DID often resemble internalized voices or dialogues and may be understood as intrusions into consciousness that are partially excluded from awareness in traumatized individuals. In BPD, auditory-verbal hallucinations are usually stress-related and strongly associated with childhood trauma [152, 153]. Nonetheless, the connection between auditory-verbal hallucinations and trauma-related intrusions is controversial and still under investigation. Recently, Pietkiewicz et al. [155] developed a codebook for assessing the complexity and content of auditory hallucinations. Based on interviews with healthcare professionals and voice hearers, several dimensions were identified, including the complexity of the content, autonomy, and influence of voices on the voice hearer. This codebook could help clinicians detect patients who may benefit from dissociation-based therapy approaches [155].

2.6.4 *Substance-Induced Dissociative States*

Substance-induced dissociative states do not only resemble the symptoms of dissociative disorders but they can also coexist with them. To diagnose a dissociative disorder, it must be ruled out that the relevant dissociative symptoms are caused exclusively by substances. At the same time, many people with dissociative disorders use alcohol and other substances to alleviate the stress associated with their symptoms or to numb trauma-related emotions and sensations [156, 157]. Research has shown that dissociative experiences can be actively induced by alcohol, barbiturates, benzodiazepines, and similarly acting hypnotics or depressant drugs [158–160]. Beta-adrenergic blockers, scopolamine, clioquinol, marijuana, and certain psychedelic drugs were also associated with dissociative symptoms [161–164]. In experimental laboratory settings, ketamine (a N-methyl-D-aspartate glutamate receptor antagonist), methylenedioxymethamphetamine (MDMA), and cannabis were found to induce dissociation [165, 166]. Findings from two recent placebo-controlled studies suggest that dissociative states increased significantly under the influence of MDMA and cannabis and to a lesser extent under the influence of cocaine [164]. Another study found that the 1-year prevalence of substance use significantly predicted dissociation in participants with active substance use, independent of childhood trauma which was also associated with higher levels of dissociation [167].

Understanding the distinction between substance-induced and disorder-related dissociation as well as their overlap is crucial in the diagnostic process. Substance-induced dissociative symptoms can range from mild depersonalization or derealization to more severe experiences like amnesia and fugue. It is therefore important to determine whether dissociative symptoms are caused directly and exclusively by substance use or whether they are part of a more complex dissociative disorder that might be exacerbated by substance use [162].

CHAPTER 3

Assessment of Dissociation and Diagnostic Process

Abstract Early detection of dissociative symptoms and disorders is important to prevent more serious chronic problems and to enable adequate treatment as early as possible. A first step towards adequate understanding and treatment is a thorough assessment of dissociation. Various self-report scales and screening questionnaires have been developed, including the Dissociative Experiences Scale (DES), Cambridge Depersonalization Scale (CDS), Dissociation Questionnaire (DIS-Q), Multiscale Dissociation Inventory (MDI), Multidimensional Inventory of Dissociation (MID), and Somatoform Dissociation Questionnaire-20 (SDQ-20). Acute dissociative states can be assessed using the Clinician Administered Dissociative States Scale (CADSS), Dissociative Stress Scale Acute (DSS-Acute), and Dissociative Symptom Scale. Following a positive screening, a clinician-administered structured interview, such as the Structured Clinical Interview for DSM–IV Dissociative Disorders (SCID-D) or the Dissociative Disorders Interview Schedule (DDIS) should be conducted by or in consultation with a clinician familiar with dissociative disorders and in a multidisciplinary team or network. During the screening and diagnostic process, both the possibility of underreporting and overreporting of symptoms should be considered. The purpose of questions should always be transparent and suggestive questions need to be carefully avoided. Guidelines recommend making clients aware of different views and opinions concerning the cause and treatment of dissociative disorders.

A. Krause-Utz, *Dissociation in Borderline Personality Disorder*,
https://doi.org/10.1007/978-3-032-06339-7_3

Keywords Assessment · Diagnostic process · Interviews · Screening · Questionnaires

Early detection of dissociative symptoms and disorders is important to prevent more serious chronic problems and to offer adequate treatment as early as possible. The heterogeneity and complexity of dissociative symptoms requires a thorough assessment with appropriate scales. Differential diagnoses pose a challenge in the diagnostic process and misdiagnoses can lead to inefficient treatment indications, delaying effective treatment for years [86, 91, 168]. According to established guidelines, a first step toward adequate understanding and treatment is a thorough assessment of dissociative states and symptoms [169, 170].

Various self-report scales, screening questionnaires, and clinician-administered structured interviews have been developed to assess the prevalence and severity of dissociation and dissociative disorders; see [170, 171]. Screening instruments can help identify people at increased risk for developing or having symptoms of a dissociative disorder. Following a positive screening for the presence of a dissociative disorder, conducting a structured interview, such as the Structured Clinical Interview for DSM–IV Dissociative Disorders (SCID-D) [172] and Dissociative Disorders Interview Schedule (DDIS) [173] is recommended.

3.1 Self-Report Scales and Screening Questionnaires

The following questionnaires were found to validly and reliably assess trait dissociation (the general tendency to experience dissociative symptoms) or acute dissociative states and are also used for research purposes [170, 171]. The Dissociative Experiences Scale (DES) is one of the most widely used instruments for assessing the general tendency to experience depersonalization, derealization, amnesia, and absorption [174]. It is available in different versions, including a revised 28-items version (DES-II) [175] and a briefer 8-item screening instrument for pathological forms of dissociation (DES Taxon) [51] that were found to have strong psychometric properties [171, 176].

Other established instruments for assessing trait dissociation are (in alphabetical order) the Cambridge Depersonalization Scale (CDS) [177], the Dissociation Questionnaire (DIS-Q) [178], the Multiscale Dissociation Inventory (MDI) [41], the Multidimensional Inventory of Dissociation (MID) [42], and the Somatoform Dissociation Questionnaire-20 (SDQ-20) [179].

Acute dissociation (depersonalization/derealization, identity confusion/alteration, and amnesia) can be assessed using the Clinician Administered Dissociative States Scale (CADSS) [180]. In a German trauma-exposed sample, the translated version demonstrated excellent internal consistency and robust convergent validity [181]. It was found to discriminate patients with dissociative disorders from patients with other psychiatric disorders and healthy subjects. With this measure, acute dissociative symptoms within the past days, within sessions, or immediately following a standard psychotherapy session can be assessed.

Similarly, the Dissociative Stress Scale Acute (DSS-Acute) and its four-item short form (DSS-4) can be administered to measure acute dissociation (depersonalization, derealization, altered sensory processing) and symptom changes over time, both in clinical and experimental research settings [182, 183]. The Dissociative Symptom Scale [184] is another instrument that measures dissociative symptoms in the past week using eight items.

A newly developed scale is the Stanford Dissociation Questionnaire (SDQ) [185]. Nine items assesses three facets of dissociation (alteration in the perception of one's mind, body, and world) and can be employed to assess either trait or state dissociation. Across three studies strong content validity, a theoretically congruent factor structure, good convergent and discriminant validity, internal consistency, and temporal stability over 1 week were found. A more detailed overview of measures can be found in systematic reviews, see [170, 171].

3.2 Clinician-Administered Structured Interviews

Among established clinician-administered structured interviews, the SCID-D [172] is considered the gold standard for diagnosing dissociative disorders and trauma-related dissociation [169]. The SCID-D is a comprehensive interview that assesses depersonalization and derealization, dissociative amnesia, identity confusion, and identity alteration. Administration typically takes 30 min to 2.5 h, depending on the presence and complexity of symptoms. The SCID-D can also help distinguish between DID and factitious disorder or malingering. The SCID-D exhibits strong psychometric properties, particularly for diagnosing dissociative disorders and differentiating them from other mental disorders, good validity, test–retest and inter-rater reliability [186].

The DDIS [173] assesses symptoms of dissociative disorders and somatic symptom disorders, childhood abuse histories, and potential differential diagnoses, such as personality disorders, major depressive disorder, substance abuse, and psychotic symptoms (positive symptoms of schizophrenia, extrasensory experiences). It is a highly structured interview that allows for the DSM diagnoses of dissociative disorders, somatic symptom disorder, BPD, and major depressive disorder. The DDIS can be administered in 30–45 min and is very reliable and valid. A self-report version (SR-DDIS) also exists [187]. A study that examined the prevalence of dissociative disorders in a private psychiatric hospital inpatient setting over a period of 9 months found very good to excellent concurrent validity for a diagnosis of DID or DDNOS using the DDIS, SCID-D, and DES-T [77].

For the dissociative subtype of PTSD, several assessments and screening instruments have been developed, including the Dissociative Subtype of PTSD Scale (DSPS), which can be administered as a self-report measure or integrated in a semi-structured interview. Fifteen items assesses current and lifetime history of dissociative symptoms with the subscales derealization/depersonalization, loss of awareness, and psychogenic amnesia [94]. The Dissociative Subtype of PTSD Interview (DSP-I) [188] is a clinician-administered interview that assesses the presence and severity of PTSD-DS symptoms, especially depersonalization and derealization. A supplementary checklist enables differentiation from other trauma-related dissociative symptoms. It showed high internal consistency, good divergent validity with scales of somatization, anxiety, and depression, and good convergent validity with relevant items of the Clinician-Administered PTSD Scale for DSM-5 (CAPS-5). The CAPS-5 is considered the gold standard in PTSD assessment, and can also be used to assess dissociative symptoms and the dissociative subtype of PTSD. It is a 30-item structured interview that determines the presence of a current or lifetime diagnosis of PTSD based on the onset, duration, and severity of symptoms and their impact on social and occupational functioning over the past week [189].

3.3 Diagnostic Process: Recommendations and Challenges

Guidelines recommend that a comprehensive and detailed diagnostic assessment is conducted by or in consultation with a clinician familiar with dissociative disorders, preferably within a multidisciplinary team or network [169, 170]. Diagnosis should preferably be based on multiple sources of information (from the patient, relatives, files etc.). The involvement of relatives and partners can be helpful but is sometimes undesirable (e.g. in cases of ongoing abuse). Therefore, these options should first be discussed with the clients and their wishes should guide the entire diagnostic process. To fully understand and assess the complexity of symptoms, a systematic assessment of the client's personal-social history is necessary. A comprehensive intake should include current complaints and symptoms, possible triggering situations and events, as well as the history of symptoms and possible treatment. It should further include a thorough mental status examination of cognitive, affective, and psychomotor functions, motivation, and impulse control. The social-personal history should be assessed in a calm, empathic, nonjudgmental, validating, and transparent manner that enables the client to identify precursors of current symptoms and to put them in a chronological perspective. Thereby, client and clinician can construct a more coherent personal narrative that helps to understand how symptoms emerged and how and why they are maintained.

During the screening assessment and diagnostic process, both the possibility of underreporting and overreporting of symptoms should be considered [169, 170]. Underreporting may be due to reduced awareness or insight, denial, and a reluctance to disclose experiences, for example, due to feelings of shame or distrust. People entering the healthcare system for the first time might find it difficult to express their experiences and often refrain from sharing dissociative experiences unless encouraged. Some people may have learned to mask, hide, deny, or minimize their symptoms because of past invalidation or because they do not know how to interpret and verbally express their experiences. Dissociative experiences are often only shared after a safe and trusting relationship has been established and enough psychoeducation has been provided. The purpose of questions should always be transparent, especially in cases involving traumatic experiences. It is important that individuals have a clear understanding of what is meant by specific questions and that they have the freedom to describe their experiences in their own language. Brand et al. [168] argue that DID is more often under-diagnosed than over-diagnosed, partly due to efforts to avoid stigma, skepticism, and lack of knowledge. Clinicians specialized in dissociative disorders point out that subtle forms of DID are more common and representative than overt manifestations, since symptoms are often masked by depression, self-harm or substance abuse; this can lead to misdiagnosis and delay diagnosis [86].

Overreporting can also have various reasons. As with any other mental disorder, intentional distortion or exacerbation of behavioural signs and symptoms, and malingering due to apparent external rewards or incentives must be ruled out during the process of diagnosing dissociative disorders [15]. However, some individuals with DID might overreport symptoms, which does not deny their existence and does not indicate malingering [190]. In this context, the possible influence of media has been discussed. Media portrayals of DID often oversimplify and dramatize identity changes and other symptoms, conveying certain stereotypes. Some people with DID may be prone to internalize these exaggerated stereotypes or come to believe that they are expected to express their symptoms in a similar way to be taken seriously [191]. While media portrayals can influence the way people understand and report dissociative symptoms, this does not negate the underlying severity of symptoms and the potential impact of trauma. Traumatic experiences are common in people with pathological dissociation, particularly complex dissociative disorders, while they are not always the direct cause. In particular, complex chronic dissociation should not be equated with other dissociative phenomena which are often caused by factors other than trauma [37, 38, 192, 193]. Suggestive questions, hinting at an unresolved trauma history, should be carefully avoided. In general, (recovered) memories should be viewed as current recollections of past events and not as a direct representation of the past. At the same time it is important not to doubt, dismiss, or invalidate these recollections, as this could be retraumatizing [86]. Instead, the subjectivity of memories should be openly discussed as a universal phenomenon of human existence.

As addressed in the next chapter, there is still some debate concerning the development of chronic complex dissociative disorders, particularly DID [37, 59, 86, 194]. Different etiological models have led to different treatment approaches. Treatment guidelines recommend that clients should be made aware of these different views and opinions (for example, the assumed role of trauma) to better understand and choose the treatment environment and approach that is most appropriate for them, while being informed about associated risks and benefits and the availability of treatments [169, 195].

CHAPTER 4

Etiological Models and Risk Factors for Dissociation

Abstract Dissociative symptoms can develop for various reasons and do not necessarily have to be pathological. The etiology of pathological dissociation and dissociative disorders typically involves a complex interplay of genetic and neurobiological vulnerabilities, temperamental predispositions, and environmental stressors, including psychological stress and trauma as well as socio-cognitive and cultural factors. Individuals with dissociative disorders report more traumatic life experiences, including child abuse and neglect. Poor stress tolerance, problems in emotion regulation, negative self-concepts, and identity disturbances may contribute to the persistence of dissociation. People with dissociative disorders often have limited awareness of their emotions and current needs, are more prone to supress emotions, and show altered self-referential processing. Deeply rooted schemas and maladaptive core beliefs may increase affective instability and interpersonal sensitivity. For some people, dissociation may be a learned strategy to cope with overwhelming experiences. However, sleep disturbances, physical exhaustion, substance use, and sensory overload can also trigger dissociation. Dissociative symptoms were further linked to neuropsychological deficits and alterations in brain networks implicated in cognitive and emotional processing. The development of chronic dissociative experiences is therefore complex and varies from person to person, depending on biopsychosocial and cultural background, co-occurring physical and mental health problems, and available support systems.

A. Krause-Utz, *Dissociation in Borderline Personality Disorder*, https://doi.org/10.1007/978-3-032-06339-7_4

Keywords Etiology · Risk factors · Trauma · Socio-cognitive model · Mechanisms

Dissociative experiences can have various causes. A complex interplay of genetic and neurobiological vulnerabilities, temperamental dispositions, and environmental stressors can predispose people to experience dissociation due to various direct and indirect influences. Chronic stress and trauma, alterations in self-referential processing, as well as social and cultural factors can contribute to the development of chronic dissociation. Internal and external triggers for acute dissociative episodes range from emotional distress, negative thoughts and memories, to sleep disturbances, and substance use; see [37, 38]. Given the broad spectrum of dissociative phenomena and disorders, it is important to consider the individual's unique biopsychosocial, cultural, and psychopathological background [37, 193, 196].

While most researchers agree that the etiology of dissociative disorders is complex, the causes of dissociative disorders, particularly DID, are still debated. Currently, there are two main perspectives in the field; for a more detailed discussion, see [37, 59, 194, 196]. In brief, trauma models emphasize the role of traumatic stress, especially childhood abuse and neglect, while socio-cognitive models focus on cognitive and temperamental dispositions (fantasy proneness, imaginative involvement, hyper-associativity), difficulties with meta-consciousness, and media influences. Amid these debates, it has been emphasized that trauma models and socio-cognitive models are not necessarily opposed [37, 38, 193]. Lynn et al. [37, 196] argue that a comprehensive account of dissociative disorders must extend beyond the reach of trauma models and socio-cognitive models [37, 196]. They call for a transtheoretical integrative perspective that considers multiple causal and influencing factors [37, 193, 196]. Similarly, Sar et al. [38, 193] argue that the possible impact of trauma on the development of dissociative disorders needs to be understood within a broader biopsychosocial framework that also encompasses sociocultural and metacognitive factors.

In the following, different theoretical perspectives that are relevant for understanding dissociation in various mental disorders, including BPD, are described. Psychological stress and trauma are important risk factors, although it is still not yet fully understood why some people experience dissociation during traumatic situations why others do not, and why some people develop dissociative disorders after trauma. Socio-cognitive factors, sleep disturbances, emotion dysregulation, and maladaptive schemas may play an important role here. Difficulties in emotion regulation, deeply rooted schemas and maladaptive core beliefs may influence how individuals who are prone to dissociation process stressful situations. Lastly, neurobiological models on dissociation and empirical evidence from psychophysiological research, and neuroimaging studies are presented. While the neurobiological underpinnings of dissociation are not yet entirely understood, neuropsychological deficits and alterations in brain networks implicated in cognitive, emotional, and self-referential processing were found in individuals with higher levels of dissociation.

4.1 Trauma-Related Dissociation

Psychological trauma is an important risk factor for dissociation. Individuals with dissociative disorders report significantly more childhood adversities, including severe abuse and neglect by primary caregivers, parental unavailability and disorganized attachment, institutional abuse (for example in foster care or orphanages), severe bullying, and painful medical interventions at a young age [197–201]. Other studies linked dissociation to adult sexual and physical violence, intimate partner violence, human trafficking, natural disasters, torture, political and mass violence, including living in dangerous war situations (civilian exposure to war and genocide). Findings have been summarized through systematic meta-analyses [197, 202] and comprehensive reviews [12, 199–201].

A comprehensive meta-analysis of 65 studies (7352 individuals) found that individuals with more severe childhood abuse and neglect report higher levels of dissociation than non-abused or non-neglected subsamples with similar sample characteristics [203]. This association was particularly strong for child sexual and physical abuse. Earlier age of onset, a longer duration of abuse, and abuse by parental figures were identified as significant moderators. Another meta-analysis [202] of 30 eligible empirical studies, comprising of 2199 clinical participants, found positive significant associations between different forms of childhood adversity and dissociation, with aggregated effect sizes in the small-to-moderate range. Some researcher have pointed out that more longitudinal prospective studies are needed since most studies included retrospective self-reports, which can be biased, see [191]. As mentioned above, the impact of trauma on the development of dissociation should be understood within a broader biopsychosocial perspective that also considers moderating and mediating factors [193].

Trauma models assume that dissociation is a natural response to overwhelming experiences [12, 54, 72]. Dissociative symptoms, such as depersonalization, derealization, and out-of-body experiences, can help cope with distressing thoughts, emotions, and sensations that are too stressful to process and that cannot be integrated into existing views of the world, other people, and oneself. Peritraumatic dissociation refers to dissociative experiences during a traumatic event. Some people may have the impression that the traumatic event is not happening to them but to someone else, or they may feel as if they are viewing themselves in the traumatic situation from a greater distance. Thereby, trauma-related emotions, thoughts, and sensations may become disconnected and may later reoccur as sudden unwanted intrusions into consciousness. Similar to traumatic situations, dissociation may then function as a self-protective mechanism to escape trauma-related emotions and memories.

It is not yet entirely clear whether trauma-related dissociation is qualitatively different from other forms of dissociation or other altered states of consciousness. While dissociative experiences are common in individuals who developed PTSD, only symptoms of derealization and depersonalization distinguished the dissociative subtype from PTSD without this subtype. Individuals with the dissociative subtype of PTSD further frequently report an altered sense of time, auditory-verbal hallucinations (voice hearing), out of body experiences, and emotional numbing [204]. Based on studies in patients with this dissociative subtype, it has been proposed that a distinct neurobiological profile of emotional overmodulation underlies these symptoms [205, 206], see Sect. 6.1.

Several theories have been proposed to explain how peritraumatic dissociation may increase the risk of developing mental disorders, such as PTSD. As described in the following sections, dissociation may lead to a dampening of autonomic arousal and a reduction in stress or fear responses, which can increase the risk that dissociation is reinforced and becomes a learned stress response [207]. Dissociation may also disturb memory consolidation—the processing and integration of traumatic experiences into autobiographical memories [208–210] or lead to negative beliefs about the self [211], which may have an impact on trauma-focused treatment [20–22].

4.1.1 Defence Cascade Model

From an evolutionary perspective, dissociation could be an important survival mechanism in threatening situations where there are imminent threats but limited opportunities for active defence or escape [61, 212, 213]. The defence cascade model conceptualizes dissociation as part of an evolutionary-based automatic response cascade that mobilizes psychobiological resources to enhance survival in life-threatening situations. According to this model, the likelihood of dissociative reactions increases with the increasing proximity of threat and with decreasing possibilities of successful defence or escape. In the face of threat, freezing responses and tonic immobility can cause the predator to lose interest and thereby increase the chance of survival. Moreover, dissociation may be accompanied by a self-protective shutdown that reduces the perception of stress and pain. This automatic self-protective reaction can help endure traumatic situations, functioning as a crucial survival mechanism. While some psychophysiological studies found a decrease in heart rate and a blunting of autonomic arousal in response to traumatic content, evidence for this model is mixed [70, 214]. In part, these inconsistencies may be explained by methodological differences including different conceptualizations of dissociation [213], see Sect. 6.3.

4.1.2 Peritraumatic Dissociation as Risk Factors for Trauma-Related Disorders

While dissociation can be highly adaptive in threatening situations, it can develop into a maladaptive coping strategy and a risk factor for trauma-related and dissociative disorders. There is evidence that individuals who experienced peritraumatic dissociation are more likely to dissociate in the presence of traumatic reminders as well as other stressors; see [12, 201, 205].

Cognitive-behavioural models assume that different learning-theoretical processes could play a role here. On the one hand, dissociation may be negatively or positively reinforced once it reduces fear or increases control and a sense of predictability or stability. Dissociation often helps endure distress and may be perceived as a shield that helps to gain inner distance and remain calm in stressful situations. This increases the likelihood that dissociation will become a habitual response to cope with distress and to avoid traumatic re-experiencing. Post-traumatic dissociation is often triggered by traumatic reminders that are subjectively associated with the past event. However, over time, dissociation can also generalize to other stressful situations and ultimately function as an escape mechanism or avoidance strategy [207, 215]. This process may be unconscious and automatic or actively self-induced, for example through self-hypnosis or substance use.

Another theory is that peritraumatic dissociation increases the risk of trauma-related disorders, because it disturbs memory consolidation and hinders the processing, integration, and contextualization of traumatic experiences [208–210]. This theory suggests that dissociation interferes with the ability to properly process and encode trauma-related experiences (emotions, thoughts, sensations, behavioural impulses), which leads to subjective memory fragmentations and the development of PTSD symptoms, including dissociative flashbacks. In other words, it is assumed that dissociation prevents the integration of memories into a coherent autobiographical narrative.

Stressful characteristics of the traumatic events are compartmentalized and stored as segregated elements in autobiographical memory that can later be reactivated through traumatic memories. Unintegrated thoughts, emotions, sensations, and behavioural impulses associated with the trauma can form an individual trauma network and recur in (dissociative) flashbacks or unwanted intrusions into conscious awareness. Flashbacks are usually accompanied by a loss of continuity in subjective experience, as if the traumatic events were happening again or repeating themselves. Based on the aforementioned defence cascade model, Schauer and Elbert [60] proposed that traumatic reminders trigger a similar cascade of fear responses as experienced during the traumatic event itself.

While individuals who experienced peritraumatic dissociation report more memory problems and memory fragmentations, evidence for disturbed memory consolidation is still mixed; according to a review of sixteen studies, findings were most consistent for subjective memory fragmentation but less clear for computer-generated or rater-coded measures of memory processing [210]. Some studies found deficits in the encoding of new information, particularly stressful material, and memory retrieval of traumatic memories, associated with altered activity in brain regions that are involved in memory consolidation, such as the hippocampus and prefrontal cortex, see [19], Sects. 5.4 and 6. Nonetheless, more research is needed to understand how dissociation affects memory processes and to identify the underlying neural mechanisms.

Another way in which peritraumatic dissociation may increase the risk of PTSD is through an increase in trauma-related perceptions and cognitions, such as feelings of hopelessness, helplessness, mental defeat, guilt, self-blame, and loss of control [211]. High levels of dissociation may increase the feeling of helplessness, guilt and self-blame, for example because dissociation is subjectively interpreted as a sign of weakness and a lack of ability to act. These trauma-related beliefs can lead to negative appraisals of the traumatic event and one's own behaviours and reactions, which are well-known risk factors for PTSD.

4.1.3 *Childhood Trauma and Developmental Aspects*

Trauma models propose that the effects of trauma-related dissociation are particularly severe and long-lasting when traumatic stress began early in life and happened during sensitive phases of psychosocial and neurobiological development. Neurobiological changes and attachment disruptions may play an important role here. Abuse by primary caregivers or other people and institutions that were supposed to provide safety and protection involves a fundamental betrayal of trust, which may lead to more profound forms of dissociation.

It is assumed that children are generally more prone to dissociation, because they still have a limited repertoire of coping strategies, greater difficulties understanding and verbalizing their experiences, and a limited ability to form a consistent sense of self that persists across different situations [106, 216, 217]. Children still need to develop a set of effective, flexible skills to handle stressful experiences. They typically rely on other people for their basic needs and are less able to actively defend themselves or escape abusive situations. Moreover, children are generally less able to fully understand and "mentalize" the motives of others, including possible reasons for inconsistent or abusive behaviour.

4.1.3.1 *Impact of Adverse Childhood Experiences on Neurobiological Development*

Early life stress leads to disruptions in the normal development of emotion regulation, self-control, and identity, which may further increase the risk that children will resort to dissociation to cope with difficult situations [106–108]. Numerous studies have shown that adverse life experiences, such as abuse and neglect, can have long-lasting effects on brain development and neurobiological processes [218, 219]. Alterations in the structure and function of brain areas implicated in stress regulation, emotion processing, and executive control can contribute to problems in self-regulation at later developmental stages [220, 221]. The development of dissociative tendencies and disorders should then be understood in a larger biosocial context, as part of an ongoing psychological and neurobiological adaptation to aversive environments. Dissociation may initially arise as a necessary adaptation to cope with the emotional distress and confusion associated with parental abuse and neglect and may later be maintained to deal with emotional and interpersonal problems in adolescence and adulthood [106–108].

4.1.3.2 Attachment

Attachment theory posits that a secure attachment to primary caregivers is crucial for developing a sense of security and stability that enables infants and children to confidently explore the world and develop trust in others [222, 223]. The bonding process between infants or children and their primary caregivers is an important part of basic psychosocial development [106, 217, 224]. Strong social support, restorative relationship experiences, and experiences of safety and predictability in close relationships are important protective factors against the development of psychopathologies after traumatic experiences [201, 225, 226].

Child abuse and neglect represent serious disruptions in the attachment process between infants or children and their caregivers [217]. Yet, insecure attachment can also arise from various other factors that compromise the caregivers′ ability to provide ongoing care and support. Negative life events such as poverty or physical and mental illnesses can overwhelm parental resources. Parents who are normally loving and caring can suddenly withdraw and become unresponsive to the child's needs and distress. In this case, the parent is both a desired source of comfort and support and a source of threat and unpredictability [217]. Children may sense the helplessness or inner conflicts of their parents and attempt to protect them by becoming overly self-reliant yet closely and anxiously attached to them, adopting a disorganized attachment style [217].

Bowlby [227] proposed that early attachment experiences serve as an internal working model for later relationships [227, 228]. When caregivers are unavailable, abusive, or inconsistent in their behaviour, the infant or child internalizes unintegrated internal working models of their relationship and develop an insecure attachment style. In adult relationships, insecurely attached people may be overly anxious or avoidant, or constantly oscillate between the need for closeness, a deep-seated fear of intimacy, and the need for self-reliance and independence [222, 229, 230]. People with such a disorganized (anxious.-ambivalent) attachment style often crave close relationships and simultaneously push other people away or avoid intimacy due to a severe fear of abandonment. When they are parents and caregivers themselves, this can contribute to the unconscious intergenerational transmission of dissociation and abuse [231]. It can create a pattern in which unresolved childhood experiences manifest as emotional withdrawal or unresponsiveness to the child's distress, which inadvertently and unintentionally harms the children [232]. While the underlying processes are not yet understood, dissociation may reactivate old attachment patterns through dissociative flashbacks or unconscious neurobiological process which overwhelm the caregiver´s resources and abilities for self-regulation and co-regulation [233]. The greater the similarity between infant or child and mother, the greater the risk of such reactivation [233].

Empirical evidence from prospective and cross-sectional observational studies supports the association between disorganized attachment and dissociative experiences, but also underlines the role of moderating and mediating factors [217, 224, 233, 234]. Children whose parents have a dissociative disorder, a history of trauma, and serious mental health problems were found to be at higher risk for experiencing dissociation themselves, due to various direct and indirect influences. A comprehensive review of prospective studies suggests that early attachment-related stressors are relevant for the development of dissociative outcomes, both in the presence or absence of maltreatment [224]. One prospective study [235] included 274 girls and boys who had experienced severe sexual abuse (41% of children were abused by a family member) and a comparison group of 150 children. Disorganized attachment (assessed through children's narratives using a story completion task) and emotion dysregulation at the initial assessment mediated the association between child sexual abuse and dissociation 1 year later. In another prospective study [231], children of insecure caregivers with unresolved loss showed more behaviour problems from middle childhood to early adolescence. However, this association was significant, even when controlling for caregiver psychopathology, suggesting that their levels of dissociation and depression did not fully explain the association between childhood abuse and dissociation. A recent scoping review of twenty studies in caregivers with BPD found some evidence for an effect of dissociation on the interactional relationship quality within parent–child dyads [233]. However, the concept of intergenerational transmission of dissociation remains difficult to define and to study. Moreover, the underlying processes are highly complex and involve various intra- and interpersonal dynamics, environmental, societal, familial, and genetic factors [217]. All these factors and processes can shape the psychosocial neurobiological development and contribute to dissociative symptoms, both in the presence and absence of parental maltreatment [217, 224].

4.1.3.3 Mentalization and Identity Formation

When their primary caregivers are abusive, this fundamental betrayal of trust can lead to negative self-attributions, maladaptive schemas, chronic shame, self-disgust, and guilt, see [236–239]. Some children may actively distance themselves from attempts to mentalize the motives of abusive and hostile caregivers, while others may try to "over-mentalize" their motives to anticipate and prevent further abuse and learn to ignore own needs and suppress difficult emotions [240]. Children often struggle to integrate conflicting positive and negative relationship experiences, which can lead to distorted representations of the self and others, as being either entirely good or being entirely bad [223]. The formation of identity can be obstructed, resulting in a fragmented scattered sense of self, self-alienation, and estrangement from others, associated with chronic dissociative experiences [236, 237].

With respect to DID, trauma models assume that childhood trauma can lead to a fragmentation of the personality into segments [241]. When this separation takes place in a highly coherent manner—through consistent rituals and symbolic mechanisms—discrete senses of self can develop that are associated with unique ways of thinking, feeling, and behaving. Over time, discrete states of consciousness are organized around a prevailing affect, sense of self, and body image, which allows some aspects of the personality to mature and intellectual, interpersonal, and artistic skills to develop, while intolerable traumatic experiences are encapsulated. Over time, these discrete states can become increasingly elaborated, ultimately resulting in dissociative self-states, as seen in DID [241].

4.1.3.4 Dissociation, Revictimization, and Intimate Partner Violence

Individuals who experienced abuse and neglect in childhood are at increased risk of becoming victims of domestic violence [242–244], physical and sexual violence/abuse by strangers, kidnapping, stalking, or crime in adulthood [235, 245–248] and there is evidence that dissociation contributes to the increased risk of revictimization [245, 249, 250].

One theory is that dissociation reduces risk perception in unsafe and abusive situations, which can lead to riskier behaviour and more difficulties perceiving and expressing boundaries in an assertive way. General difficulties in emotion regulation and impulsivity may be modulating factors [251, 252]. Dissociative experiences can go hand in hand with risky decisions and impulsive behaviours [253, 254]. Feeling detached from oneself and the environment or dissociative absorption can make it harder to become aware of the consequences of one´s actions [253, 255, 256], which may lead to more impulsive decision-making [257] and more impulse control problems [258, 259].

A combination of dissociation proneness, BPD features (affective instability, self-harming impulsivity, unstable self-image, negative relationship experiences), and maladaptive cognitive coping (self-blame, rumination, catastrophizing) linked experiences of child sexual abuse to sexual violence in intimate relationships [260].

An experimental study [30] in women with a primary BPD diagnosis—almost half of them having comorbid PTSD—found that women who reported more impulsive sex with uncommitted partners also reported more symptoms of derealization and more dissociation symptoms in sexual situations—associations which were not present in healthy participants. When exposed to an erotic narrative in a laboratory setting, an increase in acute dissociative symptoms, especially derealization and depersonalization, was found.

In a large multicentre study including $N = 2156$ college students from the Netherlands and New Zealand [245], dissociation, PTSD symptoms, trauma load, loneliness, and drug use were found to contribute to an increased risk of emotional, physical, and sexual victimization after age 14. More specifically, a data-driven theoretical path analysis revealed that childhood maltreatment was associated with cognitive-emotional patterns (anxious attachment style, emotion dysregulation), which predicted more risky sex behaviour and thereby more revictimization. While the cross-sectional design of the study limits the interpretation of findings, this study suggest that dissociation may increase the risk of revictimization when it is part of a more complex pattern of emotional-cognitive behavioural dysregulation.

When revictimization occurs in the context of intimate relationships, additional contextual and situational factors should be taking into account. Intimate partner violence (IPV) is serious global problem that affects millions of people and can take various emotional (verbal, psychological), physical, and sexual forms of abuse, violence, and coercion [261]. The interpersonal dynamics are usually very complex. Sometimes both partners engage in acts of violence against each other, for example, out of self-protection or an unconscious reactivation of past experiences of violence during dissociative flashbacks [262]. During dissociative episodes, some people may act violently without fully realizing it. It has been discussed that dissociation can lead to a disconnection from violent behaviour and to a subsequent denial or difficulty with taking responsibility [255]. Memory gaps and disconnection from painful emotions, such as fear, shame, and guilt, can make it difficult to acknowledge and take responsibility for these violent actions, increasing the risk of further acts of violence [255, 263].

Higher levels of dissociation have been associated with more violence in intimate relationships, including reciprocal IPV [255, 260, 263, 264]. Besides dissociation, maladaptive emotional coping (heavy alcohol and drug use), insecure attachment, a lack of problem-solving skills, maladaptive schemas, and mental health problems, such as depression, anxiety, and post-traumatic stress symptoms, especially avoidance, were implicated in IPV [244, 247, 265, 266]. An exploratory data-driven network analysis identified dissociation as an important bridge symptom that linked experiences of child maltreatment to IPV, even when mutual associations with maladaptive emotional coping, early maladaptive schemas (mistrust, alienation, enmeshment), attachment anxiety, social support, BPD features, and PTSD symptoms were taken into account [264]. However, the cross-sectional design of this study limits the interpretation and more longitudinal studies are needed to better understand how dissociation contributes to IPV [267]. Sociocultural and situational factors as well as reciprocal couple dynamics need to be taken into account as well. Low socio-economic status, unemployment, social isolation, societal-cultural attitudes accepting or justifying violence and aggression, and weak community sanctions health, educational, economic, and social policies or laws were found to be risk factors for IPV [244, 268,

269]. Social support, restorative relationship experiences, and community factors (access to resources and services, economic and financial help, medical care and mental health services, restraining orders and safe, stable housing) were found to be protective factors. Therefore, the role of dissociation should be understood in this broader context of IPV risk factors.

4.1.3.5 *Impact of Dissociation on Trauma-Focused Treatment*

Evidence suggests that dissociation may be a potential barrier to desired changes in information processing and memory during trauma-focused treatment, particularly in groups with complex symptom presentations [20–22]. However, the impact of dissociation on trauma-related treatment is still debated and findings are inconsistent [270].

A proposed reason for the limited effectiveness of trauma-focused interventions in individuals with high levels of dissociation is that the ability to fully process and integrate traumatic experiences may be impaired during acute dissociative states [16, 271], see [19]. Most trauma-focused treatments focus on an integration of traumatic memories into autobiographical memory and a habituation to post-traumatic stress. The core principle of these treatments is an integration of experiences and the strengthening of a stable and coherent identity. Challenging negative beliefs, unlearning old associations, and establishing new connections is crucial for this [272]. Dissociation, on the other hand, involves a disintegration of experiences. Several studies found a negative effect of acute dissociative states on a broad range of cognitive functions, including attention, memory, and learning in stressful contexts, see Sect. 5.4. There is evidence that acute dissociation can impair emotional learning and memory [16, 271, 273]. If not adequately assessed and recognized, acute dissociation might interfere with important treatment processes [20–22].

Individuals with dissociative disorders and complex PTSD showed slower improvement in dissociative symptoms and interpersonal problems. A meta-analysis concluded that clients often keep struggling with pronounced disturbances in self-organisation and dissociation after trauma-focused interventions [274]. Some studies found poorer treatment responses in patients with the dissociative subtype of PTSD and it was discussed that they might respond differently to trauma-focused treatments [205, 275]. However, studies on the influence of dissociation on the effectiveness of trauma-focused treatments have revealed contradictory results. A first meta-analysis by Hoeboer et al. [270], raised doubt on the assumption that pre-treatment dissociation has a negative effect on trauma-focused psychotherapy in patients with PTSD [270]. However, almost all studies included in this meta-analysis assessed trait dissociation before the treatment. Only one of the included studies tested whether within session dissociation moderated the treatment response; this study also provided evidence that within session acute dissociation interferes with trauma-focused treatment [20]. In this study, Kleindienst et al. [20] investigated the impact of dissociation on the effectiveness of dialectical behaviour therapy for PTSD. Patients with low state dissociation during treatment had a higher chance to show substantial improvement and this relation consistently emerged across subgroups of PTSD patients with and without co-occurring BPD. Investigating dissociation as a state made a substantial difference as improvement was only predicted by state dissociation and not by trait dissociation.

Kleindienst et al. [21] further argue that there are two opposing aspects to dissociation. On the one hand, severe dissociation can make it more difficult to achieve improvement of PTSD severity by interfering with fundamental mechanisms of change, such as emotional learning and habituation. On the other hand, higher levels of dissociation are usually related to higher levels of pre-treatment PTSD severity [12], which leaves more room for improvement [276]. These opposing aspects of dissociation may cancel each other out, unless one of these effects is statistically controlled for. It is conceivable that a negative effect of dissociation on improvement is only seen when controlled for PTSD severity. A recent study tested this hypothesis and investigated whether the efficacy of cognitive processing therapy or modified dialectical behaviour therapy for individuals with childhood-trauma-related PTSD ($N = 193$) was affected by the level of pre-treatment dissociation, when controlling for PTSD severity [21]. Patients were randomly assigned to one of these evidence-based trauma-focused treatments. It was investigated whether a significant reduction in dissociation at an early stage of treatment was beneficial for subsequent efficacy. Baseline dissociation was a negative predictor for treatment efficacy. Moreover, a successful reduction of dissociation at an early stage of treatment was beneficial for the efficacy of trauma-focused psychotherapies. The authors discuss that a possible reason for inconsistencies in previous research is that dissociation can have different effects on trauma-focused treatment depending on the complexity of trauma and psychopathology. Studies included in the meta-analysis by Hoeboer et al. [270] report relatively low mean dissociation scores and did not account for pre-treatment psychopathology [20–22]. The impact of dissociation on the change in PTSD severity may be more complex than the previous meta-analysis suggests. A new meta-analysis is currently on its way to investigate whether pre-treatment and in-session dissociation predict subsequent improvement in symptom severity related to psychological treatment while controlling for PTSD severity at baseline (Prospero ID: CRD42024468050).

4.2 Socio-Cognitive Factors

Socio-cognitive factors associated with dissociation include fantasy proneness, imaginative involvement, hyper-association, difficulties with metaconsciousness and set shifts, and neurocognitive problems in memory and attention [196, 277, 278]. Negative beliefs about emotions and a lack of mindfulness may also exacerbate dissociative symptoms [279].

Individuals with a tendency to immerse themselves in imaginative experiences were found to be more susceptible to dissociative symptoms [280]. This tendency was linked to dissociative absorption and maladaptive daydreaming, which involves a deep engagement with internal fantasies and a diminished awareness of the external world [109, 109–111]. Dissociative absorption can also be related to external sources, such as a captivating movie or book, and lead to the point of losing awareness of one's surroundings. Research suggests that individuals with high fantasy proneness and those who engage in maladaptive daydreaming are more likely to experience dissociative symptoms, including depersonalization and derealization [109, 109–111]. The link between absorption and dissociation may involve difficulties in distinguishing between real and imagined experiences, a possible reliance on dissociation as a coping mechanism to escape difficult situations or stressful emotions, and challenges with attention and cognitive control [49, 280].

Some individuals may be more prone to experiencing dissociation, potentially due to factors like personality traits, past trauma, or genetic predispositions. Research suggests a link between dissociative experiences and susceptibility to memory distortions, which may be related to the way dissociation impacts memory processing and recall, see [37, 278, 281]. Challenges in understanding and reflecting on one's own mental states can be another important factor. People with chronic dissociation often have difficulty understanding and articulating their experiences [37], see Sect. 1.4

Hyper-association refers to an increased tendency to form connections between seemingly unrelated ideas or events. Hyper-associativity in various tasks including neutral and emotional material was associated with higher levels of dissociation [282]. There was tentative evidence that cognitive problems and alexithymia explained part of the relationship between hyper-associativity and daytime dissociation and nighttime unusual sleep experiences.

The ability to flexibly switch between different cognitive or behavioural sets (set shifts) seems to be impaired in individuals with dissociative tendencies. Research suggests that individuals with high levels of dissociation experience difficulties in rapidly adjusting to new situations or mental states, potentially contributing to the experience of detachment and disconnection characteristic of dissociation. This might also be linked to problems in emotion regulation and difficulties to disengage from dissociative flashbacks, see [37]. The ability to process, integrate, and assimilate information (for example, conflicting emotions or self-referential information) may be altered in complex dissociative disorders, such as DID, which could underlie sudden shifts in affect, thoughts, and behaviours [196, 282, 283].

Earlier formulations of the socio-cognitive model argued against the crucial role of trauma in the development of DID and other complex dissociative disorders. The socio-cognitive model initially positioned itself in contrast to the trauma model, emphasizing that empirical evidence for this model primarily stems from retrospective self-reports, which can be biased, and cautioning against the subjectivity of memories including potentially false memories [191, 191, 278, 284]. It stated that media influences, one-sided beliefs about dissociative disorders, and suggestive questioning styles by practitioners causing iatrogenic harm can influence the ways how individuals with dissociative disorders express their disturbing and conflicting experiences [278, 284]. Over time, however, the socio-cognitive model has broadened its scope to acknowledge the potential role of trauma, particularly childhood trauma, in the development of dissociative disorders, including DID. While the model still emphasizes the influence of social and cognitive factors, it recognizes that trauma can be a significant precipitating factor, especially in cases of severe dissociation. At the same time, it highlights the role of moderating and mediating factors.

Several factors may contribute to the persistence of dissociative experiences in individuals with trauma histories. As discussed in the next sections, these factors include sleep disturbances, maladaptive schemas, and emotion regulation problems. Individuals with chronic mental health conditions, including dissociation and post-traumatic stress, may find it difficult to sufficiently care for themselves, to maintain a good sleep routine and regularly exercise. They may have intrusive nightmares disturbing their sleep quality, more problems regulating emotions and use dissociation-inducing substances to self-medicate and numb emotions. They may be more easily stressed or sensitive to sensory and emotional overload, and experience greater anxiety and physical exhaustion. All of these can be triggers for acute dissociative episodes [37, 38, 192, 193, 285].

4.3 Sleep-Dissociation Perspective

The sleep-dissociation perspective is a multifactorial theory based on findings that dissociative symptoms such as depersonalization and derealization often occur when sleep and waking states of consciousness overlap. Sleep deprivation and poor sleep quality, including sleep disruptions such as parasomnias and sleep paralysis, are seen as a possible causes for frequent dissociative experiences [286–290]. Sleep disruptions can either be directly or indirectly linked to persistent dissociative experiences [196]. Psychological arousal during daytime can carry over to unusual sleep experiences [288]. Highly aversive events and negative emotional states during daytime can thereby impact the sleep–wake cycle and may subsequently lead to dissociative symptoms [196]. People with frequent dissociation may have unusual sleep patterns. As mentioned before, sleep disturbances, such as intrusive nightmares and sleep avoidance, could also partly explain dissociative symptoms in individuals with mental disorders, such as PTSD and DID. In one study, the severity of traumatic experiences was found to explain a substantial part of the link between sleep and dissociative symptoms [291].

4.4 Emotion Dysregulation and Maladaptive Emotional Coping

Emotion dysregulation is a transdiagnostic feature of various mental disorders, which has been associated with higher levels of dissociation. Emotion dysregulation generally encompasses cognitive-affective aspects such as limited awareness, lack of emotional clarity, and non-acceptance of primary emotions, which can lead to shame, guilt, and anger as secondary emotions. Behavioural aspects include difficulties engaging in goal-directed behaviour and problems with impulse control under stress. Individuals who lack flexible and effective emotion regulation strategies often feel and belief that emotions are uncontrollable [292].

Emotion dysregulation can include symptoms of both under-regulation (chronic difficulty calming down in stressful situations, intense emotional reactions, lack of emotional inhibition) and emotional over-regulation (excessive suppression, emptiness, and numbing) [205, 293]. Psychometric studies found significant positive associations between dissociative experiences and difficulties in identifying emotions [294], non-acceptance of emotions, increased shame [295], rumination, catastrophizing, self-blame [29], and a lack of adaptive emotion regulation skills [296], and a lack of problem-solving skills [297]. With regard to specific emotion regulation strategies, a meta-analysis found moderate associations between dissociation and maladaptive cognitive emotion regulation (worry, rumination, and non-acceptance) as well as experiential and behavioural avoidance (thought and emotional suppression) [296]. The authors discuss that other factors probably play a modulating role in this moderate association.

Alexithymia, the diminished ability to identify and express emotional states has been moderately to strongly correlated to trait dissociation in clinical samples and non-clinical populations, see [298]. The diminished ability to identify and express emotions or bodily states may play a role in the development of chronic dissociative states [8, 31, 106, 299]. However, alexithymia is a stable cognitive state of externally oriented thinking, while dissociation is more closely related to an unstable sense of self [300].

4.5 Early Maladaptive Schemas and Schema Modes

Schemas are mental representations about oneself, the world, and others, which comprise emotions, cognitions, memories, and bodily sensations. Maladaptive schemas often develop when core emotional and psychological needs are not met due to a mismatch between a child's basic needs and their environmental resources or capacities, for example due to abuse and neglect [301], and have been associated with dissociation [265, 302, 303]. Early maladaptive schemas often centre around the need for connection, autonomy, and reasonable limits [301, 304]. A meta-analysis of nine cross-sectional studies (pooled $N = 2300$) found that dissociative symptoms were positively correlated with almost all early maladaptive schemas under investigation. Strongest associations were found with defectiveness/shame, vulnerability to harm, and social isolation schemas [305]. However, heterogeneity between studies was quite high, and it remains unclear whether early maladaptive schema are a risk factor for dissociation or a consequence [306, 307]. Early maladaptive schemas and dissociative experiences may mutually reinforce each other, worsening feelings of alienation, shame, and defectiveness. The perpetuating nature of schemas increases the risk of a vicious cycle where dissociative experiences and core beliefs influence the way current events are perceived [37, 308].

Schema modes are moment-to-moment emotional states and coping behaviours, triggered by experiences congruent with personal schemas [265, 301]. The schema-mode model proposes that reactivated schemas may partly explain the dramatic mood and identity fluctuations in people with complex dissociative disorders [301, 303]. Prominent schema modes in individuals with dissociative disorders, BPD, and avoidant personality disorder are the vulnerable child mode, dysfunctional parent modes, and avoidant coping modes [303]. These schema modes centre around early maladaptive schemas of disconnection, rejection, over-vigilance, and inhibition. It has been proposed that dissociative experiences occur as part of a detached protector mode, which helps to cut off emotional pain, shame, and guilt [304, 309].

Two studies in patients with a primary BPD diagnosis found positive correlations between dissociation (Wessex Dissociation Scale) and various schema modes. The first study found associations with the angry and impulsive child mode and the abandoned and abused child mode [302]. The other study found strong correlations with the detached protector mode, the angry and impulsive child mode, the punitive and demanding parent mode, and the vulnerable child mode [310]. These findings suggest that dysfunctional schema modes associated with defectiveness, shame, mistrust, and vulnerability to harm, are elevated in individuals with dissociative tendencies [83]. Negative self-representations implicitly related to self-rejection were also linked to dissociation in a group of individuals with adverse life experiences [83].

4.6 Dynamic Interplay of Symptoms in Psychological Network Analyses

In recent years, several studies investigated whether dissociative symptoms are part of a complex symptom matrix, considering the multivariate interplay of symptoms. Psychological network analysis, a graph-theoretical approach, is well-suited for analysing interrelations among clinical symptoms and psychosocial constructs. With this method, variables are represented as *nodes*, and their associations are represented by *edges* between the elements of a network. The structure of symptom interdependence can be calculated and visualized in a partial correlation network [311]. The method allows for the quantification of each symptom´s role within the network using centrality indices, which indicate how strongly a node is connected to others [311]. Key strengths of network analysis are its ability to generate hypotheses about the possible pathways through which symptoms interact, for example by identifying variables that connect different clusters of variables.

In one study, symptoms of BPD, PTSD, and CPTSD were assessed in a sample of 219 adults with histories of institutional child abuse and analysed using network analysis [36]. Symptoms of PTSD and CPTSD were strongly connected within disorders and to a lesser degree between disorders, while BPD symptoms were weakly connected to others. Dissociation and traumatic re-experiencing were the nodes with the highest centrality. This network analysis suggests that dissociation is one of the central symptoms that might be an important target for interventions in individuals with childhood adversities.

Another network analysis estimated how diagnostic criteria of BPD and PTSD are interrelated. Dissociation, feelings of detachment, and self-aggression, as well as chronic feelings of emptiness were the nodes with the highest influence overall and connected the BPD-network and the PTSD-network. This finding suggests that dissociation, detachment, inner emptiness, and self-aggression could potentially perpetuate the manifestations of occurring BPD and PTSD [35].

As mentioned before, one exploratory data-driven network analysis also showed that dissociation is an important bridge symptom that may link experiences of child maltreatment to adult IPV, when accounting for the mutual associations with maladaptive emotional coping, early maladaptive schemas (mistrust, alienation, enmeshment), attachment anxiety, social support, BPD features, and PTSD symptoms [264].

One network analysis in 376 health service users in Hong Kong (43.3% with pathological dissociation) investigated the relationship between BPD features, trauma, and dissociation, controlling for general non-specific mental health distress. The partial correlation network showed that dissociative experiences were associated with the BPD features impulsivity, identity disturbance, and suicidal/self-mutilation behaviour, but not with interpersonal problems [34].

Another network analysis explored associations between dissociative experiences (depersonalization derealization, amnesia, absorption), BPD features (affective instability, identity diffusion, self-harming impulsivity, and negative relationships), and childhood trauma (emotional, physical, and sexual abuse, emotion, and physical neglect) in an international sample of 921 individuals [33]. In the partial correlation network, dissociative experiences were predominantly connected to the BPD features. More specifically, depersonalization derealization was connected to affective instability and identity disturbances, dissociative amnesia was connected to self-harm, while dissociative absorption was linked to identity disturbance. A unique association between (amnestic) dissociation and neglect was observed. These findings suggest that dissociative experiences are closely linked to BPD features, also when associations with childhood trauma are taken into account.

4.7 Ecological Momentary Assessment of Dissociation in Everyday Life

Several studies used ecological momentary assessment (EMA) to monitor dissociative symptoms in everyday life. The frequency and intensity of acute dissociation was positively correlated with subjective affective arousal and this association was more pronounced in patients with a primary BPD diagnosis compared to patients with a diagnosis of major depression or panic disorder and healthy participants [182, 312, 313]. A recent EMA study in patients with a BPD diagnosis ($N = 42$) found higher levels of affective arousal, negative affective valence, and dissociation, compared to patients with depressive disorders ($N = 40$) and non-clinical controls ($N = 39$). All participants were asked to report their symptoms in smartphone-based diaries every 15 min for 13 h within a single day [312]. Dynamic structural equation modelling showed that in the BPD group, arousal and subsequent dissociation were significantly linked implying that momentary arousal above a person's daily average is followed by higher dissociation around 15 min later. Some patients with BPD further reported less negative affective valence following dissociation, which may indicate a relief from distress.

Recently, one study combined momentary assessments with the network approach [314]. Symptoms associated with BPD (including dissociation), depression, and anxiety were assessed in 37 undergraduate students over the course of 40 days. Following baseline assessment, participants answered an online survey of current symptoms twice daily. Multilevel time-series network analysis was conducted to examine how symptoms reinforced each other over time In a BPD symptom network, dissociation exerted the strongest overall influence. Momentary interpersonal difficulties predicted dissociation, which in turn predicted subsequent affective fluctuations at the within-person level. These findings suggest that interpersonal situations may play an important role in triggering dissociation and that affective arousal does not only predict but also follow dissociation.

CHAPTER 5

Experimental and Neuropsychological Research on Dissociation

Abstract Several studies used experimental designs to investigate the impact of dissociation under controlled laboratory conditions. Compared to the extensive literature on dissociative disorders and the dissociative subtype of PTSD, research explicitly focusing on dissociation in BPD is still scarce. Recent findings point to stronger increases in dissociative states after experimental stress induction in individuals with BPD compared to other clinical groups. Chronic dissociative experiences were further associated with pain hyposensitivity and altered body perception, including reduced body ownership and body connection. Neuropsychological studies in BPD found deficits in various executive functions, such as attention, memory, and emotional learning. Individuals with BPD showed impaired working memory performance when emotional distractors were presented, which was linked to acute dissociation. Moreover, cognitive control of negative words and emotional learning were impaired in BPD patients with acute dissociation. In general, neuropsychological research in groups with high levels of dissociation revealed inconsistencies. While the majority of studies found neurocognitive deficits, some studies observed no objective impairments or even enhanced performance, depending on the investigated neuropsychological domain, the operationalization of dissociation, and sample characteristics. A clearer distinction between trait and state dissociation may contribute to a more precise understanding of associated neuropsychological deficits.

A. Krause-Utz, *Dissociation in Borderline Personality Disorder*, https://doi.org/10.1007/978-3-032-06339-7_5

Keywords Cognitive functioning · Executive functioning · Experimental research · Neuropsychological research · Memory

Several studies have used experimental designs to study the impact of dissociation under controlled laboratory conditions. So far, experimental research explicitly focusing on dissociation in BPD is relatively sparse compared to the extensive literature on dissociative disorders and the dissociative subtype of PTSD. In the following, recent studies identified through systematic searches in scientific databases, including PsychInfo, PubMed, Web of Science, and the Cocrane database are described. This search also included neurobiological (neuroimaging, neurophysiological, neuropsychological, and psychophysiological) research, using combinations of relevant keyword groups. The search was limited to articles published in English, in peer-reviewed journals, described studies in human participants and used validated standardized self-report measures of dissociation.

5.1 Impact of Stress

Several experimental studies investigated how dissociative states and traits are linked to increases in acute stress in BPD [259, 315, 316]. Two studies used the Trier Social Stress Test (TSST) as a laboratory stress induction. In the first study, patients with BPD ($N = 24$) or PTSD ($N = 20$) or depressive disorder ($N = 84$) and non-clinical controls ($N = 44$) performed the TSST compared to a placebo version [315] Acute dissociation, assessed with the DSS-4, increased after the TSST stress induction, which was more pronounced in patients with BPD compared to the other groups. The BPD group reported higher levels of baseline dissociation, which predicted stronger increases in acute derealization symptoms and somatoform dissociation.

In the second study, changes in acute dissociation (DSS-4 scores) after the TSST were assessed in a sample of 51 adolescents and young adults (aged 15–25 years), who either showed above-threshold BPD ($\geq$ 5 criteria; $N = 27$) or subthreshold BPD (3–4 criteria; $N = 24$). State dissociation increases after the TSST were associated with stress, PTSD severity, and depressive symptoms, while no association between stress and trait dissociation was found [316]. Another experimental study investigated changes in acute dissociation (DSS-4) after the Mannheim Multicomponent Stress Test (MMST), which involves a simultaneous exposure to multiple stressors. Patients with BPD ($N = 29$) were compared to patients with ADHD ($N = 28$) and healthy controls ($N = 30$) [259, 317]. Again, stronger increases in dissociation after stress induction was found in the BPD group compared to the other groups.

Another study by Chung et al. [26] used a script-driven imagery approach to induce acute stress based on personal narratives [26]. Patients with a current BPD diagnosis ($N = 25$) were compared to participants with a former BPD diagnosis in remission (BPDr: $N = 20$) and healthy controls ($N = 24$). Participants were asked to vividly recall a stressful experience in their past or a neutral experience. Patients with a current BPD diagnosis reported the highest levels of dissociation, followed by rBPD participants and healthy controls. In the stressful script condition, both clinical groups showed an increase in acute dissociation. Overall, these findings support the strong association between subjective stress and acute dissociative states, especially in patients with BPD.

5.2 Pain Processing and Self-Injury

Stress-related states of dissociation were further linked to reduced pain perception in patients with a current BPD diagnosis [26, 28, 318]. The script-driven imagery study by Chung et al. [26] assessed pain sensitivity in terms of heat pain thresholds (HPT, compared to warm perception thresholds) next to dissociation during the stress condition compared to a neutral script condition. In the stressful script condition, increases in acute dissociation and higher HPT were found in patients with a current and former BPD diagnosis. Severity of trait dissociation was significantly correlated with pain hyposensitivity in those with a current BPD diagnosis, but not in the remitted group. While dissociation proneness was enhanced in both groups, it was only related to pain hyposensitivity in those with a current BPD diagnosis. Stress-related analgesia has been linked to a stronger urge to self-harm in BPD [27]. Self-harm is more prevalent in groups with chronic dissociation, which may have different reasons [29, 256, 319]. Non-suicidal self-injury is often used as a dysfunctional coping strategy to reduce distress, to deal with interpersonal conflicts, to escape painful emotions, to signal need for support, but also to terminate unwanted dissociative states [320, 321]. One study suggests that trait dissociation, self-blame, catastrophizing, and the severity of BPD features linked traumatic childhood experiences to self-harm, including suicidal behaviour and non-suicidal self-injury [29].

5.3 Body Perception

Another line of experimental research linked higher levels of dissociation to a alterations in body perception, including a stronger illusion of body plasticity [24], reduced body ownership (impression that one´s body parts do not belong to oneself) [25], and reduced body connection (awareness, integration, and utilization of one's own bodily signals) [322].

One experimental study induced the impression of body plasticity using the so-called rubber hand illusion paradigm which creates the impression that an artificial limb is part of one´s body [24]. Dissociation was associated with a stronger illusion of body plasticity, both in patients with a current or former BPD diagnosis ($N = 53$) and healthy controls ($N = 25$), even when taking BPD symptom severity into account.

In another study, body ownership experiences for 25 body areas were assessed in patients with a current BPD diagnosis ($N = 26$) or former BPD diagnosis ($N = 22$) and healthy controls ($N = 21$). Body ownership was significantly reduced in patients with a current diagnosis compared to the healthy control group. This was significantly correlated to higher trait dissociation (DES), while controlling for other BPD symptoms [25].

Another study from this research group assessed the experience of a gentle touch on one´s hands, which is usually experienced as pleasant, in 25 patients with BPD compared to 25 healthy participants. Acute dissociative experiences and affect-modulated acoustic startle response as a physiological correlate of affective processing were assessed. Patients with BPD perceived the touch as rougher, firmer, and less pleasant, regardless of the perceived intensity of the touch. A more negative evaluation of touch was associated with a stronger increase in body-related dissociative experiences after the stimulation [323].

Adding to these experimental findings, a recent study that collected self-reports in large samples from Germany ($N = 800$) and Chile ($N = 519$) found that subjective body connection (body awareness and body dissociation) could be an important link between early trauma and impairments in personality functioning [322]. Severity of childhood trauma was strongly associated with impaired personal functioning, and this association was largely explained by body dissociation.

These findings provide empirical support for alterations in body image and perception in individuals with frequent dissociative experiences. More severe dissociative experiences are related to a stronger impression that parts of the own body do not belong to oneself and an altered processing of both aversive and normally pleasant somatosensory stimuli (pain and pleasant touch). Findings particularly underscore the need for interventions targeting the awareness of bodily signals in individuals with traumatic childhood trauma and recurrent dissociation. It is also important to better understand how altered body perceptions may underlie acute dissociative symptoms of derealization and depersonalization in sexual situations in BPD. As mentioned before, an experimental study in women with a primary BPD diagnosis found that women who reported more impulsive sex with uncommitted partners also reported more symptoms of derealization and more dissociation symptoms in sexual situations—associations which were not present in healthy participants [30].

5.4 Neuropsychological and Cognitive Functioning

A growing number of studies has investigated if individuals with high dissociation proneness or dissociative disorders show cognitive deficits in certain neuropsychological domains. The majority of studies in groups with pathological dissociation found deficits in various executive functions, such as attention, working memory, immediate and delayed verbal and visual memory, autobiographical memory, and episodic memory, see [324]. Among others, one study in BPD found deficits in various neuropsychological domains, including working memory, attention, long-term verbal memory, and executive functioning [325]. However, some studies observed no cognitive deficits or even improved neuropsychological functioning [324, 326], possibly due to lower levels of dissociative pathology [326]. Differences in study designs, sample characteristics, and neuropsychological tasks may partly explain these discrepancies. Dissociation may have a more detrimental effect on neuropsychological performance in clinical groups. Healthy individuals with high dissociation proneness showed better verbal working memory [56, 327], enhanced attentional control [57] and a better ability to switch between tasks [82]. It has been proposed that a non-clinical dissociative information processing style may even be helpful for directing and dividing attention

[57, 327]. On the other hand, some studies in healthy individuals with high dissociation proneness also found impaired divided attention [328] and poor verbal memory [329]. Moreover, studies in clinical groups, such as DID patients, found both impaired working memory [283] and improved working memory [330], as well as intact working memory capacity [291]. Different conceptualizations of dissociation and study materials may also have contributed to inconsistent results.

5.4.1 *Neutral Versus Emotional Material*

Some studies used neutral task material and assessed cognitive performance in relatively stress-free experimental contexts, while others investigated neuropsychological functioning in emotional contexts using aversive material (negative pictures or words). Studies that assessed inhibitory control of negative material in the context of an Emotional Stroop Task [273] or Flanker Task [331] found an impact of emotional material on performance. Patients with DID showed impaired inhibitory control in an anxiety-provoking context [332] but not for neutral material [331, 331]. Patients with BPD showed prolonged reaction times and more errors when emotional material was presented during a working memory task [333–335] and this was linked to acute dissociation [16, 334]. Moreover, BPD patients with acute dissociation showed impaired cognitive control of negative versus neutral words [273]. Overall, the emotional valence of study material may play a role in inconsistent findings regarding neurocognitive deficits in people with dissociative disorders. There is evidence that individuals with dissociative tendencies show altered processing of emotional salient stimuli, possibly due to a heightened sensitivity to threat. Nonetheless, some inconsistencies remain, see [324].

5.4.2 *Research on Inter-Identity Amnesia in DID*

A specific line of research investigated whether patients with DID with amnesia for autobiographical details (inter-identity amnesia) show related impairments on an experimental tasks [336, 337]. In a study by Huntjens et al. [336], no objective deficits pointing to impaired transfer of information between identities was found in patients who subjectively reported amnesia for the autobiographical details included in a concealed information task. The recognition of autobiographical material was not impaired [336]. These findings suggest that subjective disturbances in episodic memory do not necessarily translate into objective memory problems in experimental tasks [336, 337]. Inter-identity amnesia in DID may include subjective avoidance of traumatic autobiographical memories [336, 337], possibly due to metacognitive deficits in allocating self-relevance to memories incoherent with one's self-view [338]. A recent study by Dimitrova et al. [339] investigated inter-identity amnesia in individuals with DID using self-relevant, subject specific stimuli, and behavioural and neural measures [339]. In line with the aforementioned studies, there was no evidence for inter-identity amnesia based on objective task outcomes. However, compared to healthy controls, patients with DID showed faster reaction times to trauma-related identity words compared to non-self-relevant trauma-related words, suggesting increased cognitive control over self-relevant trauma-related knowledge processing in DID.

5.4.3 *Research on the Impact of Acute Dissociation*

So far, most experimental neuropsychological studies conceptualized and operationalized dissociation as a general tendency to experience dissociation and investigated associations between trait dissociation and neuropsychological performance. Only few studies directly investigated the impact of acute dissociative states on neuropsychological functioning. One study in healthy individuals induced dissociation using a mirror-gazing paradigm and found impaired working memory as well as a deterioration in word recall [340]. A study by Ebner-Priemer et al. [18] compared groups of BPD patients with and without acute peri-experimental dissociation and healthy participants during an aversive differential delay conditioning procedure. Those with acute dissociation showed diminished acquisition of differential aversive delay conditioning, in terms of skin conductance responses and valence and arousal ratings to the conditioned stimulus [271]. Another study in BPD found impaired learning for aversive versus neutral stimuli during an operant conditioning task, although reversal learning was not associated with acute dissociation [341]. Two neuroimaging studies used script-driven imagery to induce acute dissociation in patients with BPD before neuropsychological task performance was assessed. In the script-driven imagery paradigm, participants prepare a personal narrative of dissociative experiences in a (non-trauma-related) past situation. Afterwards, they are asked to listen back to this script and recall their experiences as vividly as possible. A control group is asked to prepare a neural script. The first study investigated task performance and neural activity during an Emotional Stroop Task (EST) in women with BPD exposed to a dissociation-inducing script compared to BPD patients and healthy controls with a neutral script [17]. The BPD group without acute dissociation showed behavioural performance comparable to that of healthy controls, while those who recalled a dissociation script showed slower and less accurate responses. Patients who experienced acute dissociation also showed impaired interference inhibition for negative versus neutral words, which was associated with increased activity in the left inferior frontal gyrus and less activity in occipital-parietal cortices.

The second study investigated the impact of acute dissociation on neural activity and working memory performance during a modified Sternberg Task (Emotional Working Memory Task) [16]. Trials including social-affective interference (distracting pictures of interpersonal violence) were compared to trials with neutral interpersonal scenes and distractor-free working memory trials. The group of patients, who had listened back to their dissociation script, showed overall working memory impairments (across different task conditions) compared to BPD patients and healthy controls with a neutral script. Interestingly, patients with BPD also showed a deactivation in the amygdala during acute dissociation, which may suggest a stronger detachment from distressing images and simultaneous disengagement from the task. Shifting attention away from stressful images may have led to poorer task performance. In line with this idea, patients also showed reduced activity in the cuneus, lingual gyrus, and posterior cingulate—brain areas that have been implicated in visual and self-referential processing.

These findings suggest a detrimental effect of acute dissociation on emotional learning (the acquisition of paired stimuli associations in an aversive context), working memory, and inhibitory control in individuals with a primary BPD diagnosis [16, 271, 273, 341]. A clearer distinction between trait dissociation (general dissociative tendencies) and acute dissociative states may contribute to a more precise understanding of their effects on neuropsychological functioning.

CHAPTER 6

Possible Neurobiological Underpinnings of Dissociation

Abstract Neurobiological models of dissociation, such as the defence cascade model and the cortico-limbic disconnection model, propose that dissociation is associated with a blunting of autonomic arousal and increased prefrontal control of limbic activity. Over time, these models have been revised and extended to account for the dynamic interplay of large-scale brain networks and brain stem regions. Neuroimaging studies have provided evidence for alterations in dorsomedial and dorsolateral prefrontal cortical brain areas, superior frontal regions, (anterior) cingulate, posterior association areas, and basal ganglia in individuals with high levels of dissociation. Findings suggest that dissociation is associated with alterations in brain networks implicated in emotion processing, cognitive control and arousal modulation, self-referential processing, interoception, body representation, and the filtering, processing, and integration of sensory input. However, results are still quite diverse, cover a wide range of clusters in the brain, and could not always be replicated. Findings from psychophysiological studies have been mixed and mostly inconclusive. Associations with dissociation may be non-linear and the effects of different dissociative symptoms in specific diagnostic groups should be investigated more closely. State and trait dissociation may have different or even opposite neurobiological correlates which needs to be investigated more closely.

A. Krause-Utz, *Dissociation in Borderline Personality Disorder*,
https://doi.org/10.1007/978-3-032-06339-7_6

Keywords Brain · Magnetic resonance imaging · Neuroimaging · Psychophysiology · Neurobiology

Changes in psychophysiological reactivity, hormone systems, and brain structure and function might be neurobiological underpinnings of dissociation. While research in the field is steadily growing, the precise neurobiological underpinnings of dissociation are not yet fully understood. Based on neuroimaging findings in groups with high levels of dissociation or dissociative disorders, several neurobiological models and theories have been developed and are currently tested, scrutinized, and revised. In the following, empirical evidence for and against these models is described.

6.1 Models

The defence cascade model postulates that dissociation is part of an evolutionary-based automatic response cascade that mobilizes psychobiological resources in threatening situations [61, 213, 342]. According to this model, the likelihood of dissociative reactions increases with increasing proximity of the threat and with decreasing possibilities of successful defence or escape [60]. A series of steps is thought to activate distinctive psychophysiological patterns [213, 343]. *Arousal* activates the defence cascade, followed by defence *flight or fight* responses which involve sympathetic activation. A shift from sympathetic activation to parasympathetic activation is assumed to take place when defence responses have failed or become limited. The organism is assumed to fall into a parasympathetically dominated shut-down, characterized by *freezing*, *tonic immobility,* and *collapsed immobility*. It is assumed that these responses usually subside once the danger is over and that the latest stage of *quiescent immobility* is a state of rest that promotes healing [61, 213, 342]. Each of these defence reactions is assumed to activate a distinctive neural pattern, mediated by a common neural pathway that involves the amygdala, periaqueductal grey, sympathetic and vagal nuclei, and hypothalamus [61, 205]. The same cascade of fear responses may be reactivated when the individual is re-exposed to internal and external triggers associated with the threatening event in the past, resulting in dissociative flashbacks and intrusions. As mentioned below, evidence for this model is mixed, but it has strongly influence the development of other models and research in the field. While the existence of fight, flight, and freeze responses is well-established in animal and human research and recent studies found an inverted U-shaped relationship between acute dissociation and psychophysiological arousal [342], there seems to be high inter-individual and intra-individual variability in how people experience and respond to the defence cascade [214].

Neuroimaging studies point to a complex interplay of brain regions involved in arousal modulation, fear and stress reactions, self-referential processing, and emotion regulation. Based on early findings in patients with depersonalization disorder, a cortico-limbic disconnection model was proposed [344, 345]. This model suggests that a shutdown of autonomic arousal, accompanied by increased prefrontal inhibition of limbic activity, underlies symptoms of dissociation, particularly depersonalization and derealization. The amygdala is critically involved in the bottom-up-directed initiation of stress relations and fear responses, but also plays an important role in salience detection [346, 347]. Medial and dorsolateral prefrontal cortices are implicated in top-down regulatory processes such as cognitive control and arousal modulation and can dampen amygdala activity both directly and indirectly via the anterior cingulate cortex [347–349].

Based on later empirical findings in patients with the dissociative subtype of PTSD, Lanius et al. [205] proposed that increased frontal activity (in dorsal/rostral anterior cingulate cortex and medial prefrontal cortex) and reduced activity in the amygdala and insula characterize the dissociative subtype of PTSD and distinguish it from PTSD without the dissociative subtype [205]. In several neuroimaging studies from this research group, patients with and without the dissociative subtype of PTSD showed opposite patterns of brain activity in these fronto-limbic circuits [343]. While PTSD is generally associated with attentional threat biases, individuals with the dissociative subtype are thought to preferentially exhibit passive defence responses, such as tonic immobility, emotional shutdown, and compartmentalization, associated with decreased sympathetic nervous system activity [205, 206].

More recent adaptations of this model also consider the dynamic interplay of large-scale networks such as the default mode network, central executive network, and salience network, and the role of brain stem regions. Increased top-down directed activity from ventromedial prefrontal regions to subcortical areas may be implicated in increased arousal modulation during dissociation, while bottom-up directed connections from the periaqueductal grey via the amygdala to the ventromedial cortex may underlie other PTSD symptoms, such as hyperarousal [350]. Patients with the dissociative subtype of PTSD showed increased activation within emotion regulation regions, whereas patients without this subtype had increased activity in the amygdala, globus pallidus, and motor/somatosensory regions, accurately predicting the classification of the two PTSD subtypes compared to healthy controls [351]. More recently, it was proposed that altered activity and functional connectivity of (extended) midbrain and brainstem regions, such as the thalamus, periaqueductal grey, and superior colliculus [352], and altered intra- and inter-network connectivity of the default mode network and central executive network [353] may underlie recurrent depersonalization and derealization in patients with the dissociative subtype of PTSD. In summary, alterations in neural circuits implicated in filtering and integrating sensory as well as self-referential and emotional information processing have been associated with the dissociative subtype of PTSD.

For DID, Reinders et al. [355] proposed differing neural network patterns for hypo-aroused and hyper-aroused states. Dissociative states are assumed to be associated with decreased activation in the striatum/basal ganglia and hyperactivity of the prefrontal cortex, the cingulate, posterior association areas and para-hippocampal gyri [354, 355]. In a self-reported hypo-aroused (dissociative) identity state, individuals with DID activated prefrontal cortical areas and clusters in the cingulate, posterior association areas, and para-hippocampus, whereas hyper-aroused states activated the amygdala, insula, and dorsal striatum [355].

6.2 Neuroimaging Research

The aforementioned models are increasingly being tested, questioned, and revised. Rapid developments in neuroimaging techniques and analyses tools have constantly led to increased knowledge and new hypotheses in the field. Techniques, such as positron emission tomography (PET), functional and structural magnetic resonance imaging (fMRI, sMRI), magnetic resonance spectroscopy (MRS), and diffusion tensor imaging (DTI) have long been used to study brain function and structure. With MRS, concentrations of neurochemical metabolites like N-acetylaspartate (NAA), glutamate, lactate, or choline can be assessed in certain brain regions. With fMRI, changes in blood-oxygen-level-dependent (BOLD) signal (hemodynamic responses) during symptom provocation or resting-state can be detected. During resting-state, participants are asked to close their eyes or fixate on a cross, and are instructed to think of something specific. In combination with pharmacologic challenge, neuroimaging can be used to study associated alterations in neural circuits. Other studies used experimental tasks or showed aversive images during the scanning procedure and compared groups with high levels versus low levels of dissociation.

Patterns of brain activity and coactivity (functional connectivity) during experimental tasks or resting-state (in the absence of experimental stimulation) can be analysed and compared between groups and/or different time points within the same individuals. This way, alterations in dynamic large-scale networks can be analysed as well [348]. Structural MRI and DTI can be used to detect anatomical abnormalities in grey or white matter volumes. Methods in this field are rapidly evolving and the continuous development of new scanning and analysis techniques allows an increasingly better and more precise detection of alterations in brain structure and function. Some studies also used electroencephalography (EEG) to investigate associations with dissociation, but the number of studies is still limited [70, 356].

A systematic review of 33 functional and structural neuroimaging studies by Lotfinia et al. [357] aimed to identify possible transdiagnostic markers of pathological dissociation. Across different disorders, alterations in frontal and temporal regions were identified. However, findings were very diverse and spread across large clusters. Lotfinia et al. [357] concluded from their review that the robustness and generalizability of findings should be interpreted with caution due to methodological limitations, such as small or modest sample sizes [357].

Another comprehensive systematic review by Roydeva and Reinders from 2020 broadened the scope to psychophysiological (genetic) and psychobiological biomarkers, next to possible neurofunctional and neurostructural correlates of pathological dissociation across different disorders [70]. Findings from 205 unique studies were systematically reviewed. From this literature review, it was concluded that various regions in the (pre)frontal cortex may be possible neurofunctional biomarkers of pathological dissociation. More specifically, increased activity in the inferior frontal gyrus, middle frontal gyrus, and superior frontal gyrus was associated with pathological dissociation. Several studies also found altered activity in parietal regions, the(anterior) cingulate and insula, and the basal ganglia, particularly in the striatum. For the motor cortex, a slight tendency for decreased activations was observed, but these deactivations were rather widespread across primary and sensory motor cortex and pre-central gyrus. Some studies found deactivation in the amygdala, particularly in patents with BPD and PTSD, but this was not consistent across different disorders and study paradigms, requiring further study. As discussed below, more recent studies provided stronger evidence for associations between dissociation and amygdala activity [358].

With regard to brain structure, Roydeva and Reinders [70] identified volume reductions in the thalamus, basal ganglia, and hippocampus as potential neurostructural biomarkers of pathological dissociation. These brain areas are implicated in sensory processing, motor movements, procedural and conditional learning, and a variety of cognitive functions, such as autobiographical memory.

For the hippocampus, several studies also found neurofunctional alterations, both in terms of increased and decreased activity, see [70]. A recent study found an anti-correlation between resting-state functional connectivity of the right-lateralized anterior middle frontal gyrus and the right hippocampus depending on the severity of childhood trauma [359]. Findings could point to a frontal inhibition of hippocampal activity, possibly related to an attentional shift that helps avoid trauma-related self-generated thoughts.

Roydeva and Reinders [70] also looked at other neurobiological measures, concluding that decreased tumor necrosis factor alpha (TNF-α) and increased oxytocin and prolactin may be potential psychobiological biomarkers of dissociation. They recommend the investigation of immunological markers in dissociative disorders as an important avenue for future research. Genetic findings were inconclusive [360]. While some studies found associations between dissociation and polymorphisms in different single genes, no overlap between the studies was found and findings were difficult to compare. One interesting stand-alone finding from a whole blood gene expression profile analysis in patients with BPD was a positive correlations between dissociation levels and the expression of genes involved in immune system regulation (interleukin-6) as well as cellular signalling/second-messenger systems [360]. Major limitations of the study were the possibly heterogeneous cell proportions in whole blood and the heterogeneous medication.

In general, studies included in these reviews were very heterogeneous with respect to study procedure (resting-state versus task-related fMRI etc.), sample characteristics (gender, comorbidities, trauma history, medication status etc.), measures of dissociation, and analysis techniques [357, 357]. This vast heterogeneity makes it difficult to compare and integrate findings, which still varied considerably. Given the wide range of dissociative symptom, it is unlikely that their neural correlates can be confined to a few localized brain regions [357]. Depending on the symptom constellation, dissociation probably corresponds to differential neural signatures that might vary between diagnostic groups.

When divided into different diagnostic categories, Lotfinia et al. [357] found the closest overlap for PTSD and DID samples, with most consistent alterations in frontal and temporal areas. More specifically, Roydeva and Reinders [70] found overlapping neural patterns of hyperactivity in prefrontal cortical areas, the cingulate, posterior association areas, and para-hippocampal gyri in both PTSD and DID [70]. Hippocampal volumes were found to be smaller in DID and this was correlated with more dissociative amnesia [361].

For BPD, one of the most consistent neurofunctional findings is enhanced activity in the inferior frontal gyrus. Several studies found increased activity in temporal areas (inferior, middle, and superior temporal gyrus) and decreased activity in temporo-occipital regions (fusiform gyrus, cuneus, lingual gyrus), posterior cingulate, precuneus, and the amygdala [10]. Again, findings are still diverse and need to be replicated. Conceptual differences and methodological differences in the assessment of dissociation hinder a straightforward interpretation and comparison of studies.

State and trait dissociation may have different or even opposite biological correlates when evaluated independent of dissociative pathology and research paradigm [70]. Only few studies so far investigated the impact of acute dissociation, for example, using script-driven imagery or pharmacological agents and findings are still diverse [16, 28, 273, 362]. Among the first studies, Ludäscher et al. [28] assessed brain activity and pain processing during acute dissociation in a group of fifteen patients with a primary BPD diagnosis (ten of them also having PTSD) [28]. Dissociative psychopathology was associated with increased activity in the left superior frontal gyrus and decreased activity in the right middle and inferior temporal gyrus. In a subgroup of participants with comorbid PTSD, increased activity in the left cingulate gyrus was found during script-induced dissociation. Higher dissociation scores were related to increased activity in the right and left insula and reduced activity in the right parahippocampal gyrus. However, the sample size was small and a comparison group was lacking. As mentioned before, two studies combined script-driven imagery with inhibitory control tasks (Emotional Stroop Task and Emotional Working Memory Task) [16, 17]. Although the two tasks are not directly comparable, a relatively consistent finding was increased inferior frontal gyrus activity and decreased activity in occipital-parietal cortices. Patients with acute dissociation also showed reduced amygdala activity during the more distressing Emotional Working Memory Task, which included highly aversive images depicting interpersonal threat [16].

Mertens et al. [362] used script-driven imagery to induce post-traumatic dissociation through the recall of traumatic (as opposed to neutral) autobiographical memories in 51 patients with PTSD and a history of interpersonal childhood trauma [362]. During trauma recall, enhanced activity in the cerebellum, occipital gyri, supramarginal gyrus and amygdala was found. While trauma recall induced dissociation, no significant correlation with any of the observed neural alterations was found. Another study by this research group investigated brain activity during script-driven imagery compared to a within-participant, placebo-controlled pharmacological challenge paradigm (4.0 mg reboxetine versus placebo) in 47 patients with PTSD and a history of interpersonal childhood trauma [363]. Self-reported dissociation increased significantly during trauma (as opposed to neutral) script recall but did not differ between pharmacological conditions. In both conditions, trauma recall was associated with increased activity in the middle occipital gyrus and supramarginal gyrus.

In another study, the administration of a dissociation-inducing drug (ketamin) did not lead to the hypothesized increase of resting-state connectivity between amygdala and medial prefrontal regions but instead to a stronger decrease in resting-state connectivity [166]. Levels of dissociation induced in these studies were relatively low and possibly not comparable to other studies. While these researchers raised doubts on the suggested role of the amygdala in dissociative processing of trauma memories [362, 363], another recent study provided support for this idea [358].

Including a large sample of individuals with adverse childhood experiences ($N = 141$; $N = 105$ of them having clinical diagnoses, such as PTSD, depressive disorder, and somatic symptom disorder), Seitz and colleagues investigated different predictors of amygdala reactivity to social threat [358]. Participants underwent fMRI during an emotional face–matching task and completed various clinical questionnaires, including a scale on the timing, duration, and types of childhood maltreatment (abuse and neglect) and a scale on trait dissociation (German extended version of the DES). Predictors for amygdala reactivity to threat were investigated using a machine learning-based model comparison procedure that considers different possible prediction models. In this transdiagnostic sample, neither type nor timing or duration of childhood maltreatment predicted amygdala reactivity to interpersonal threat. Instead, trait dissociation clearly emerged as a strong predictor of blunted bilateral amygdala response and a possible mediator between childhood maltreatment severity and amygdala function. These findings support the idea that dissociation is associated with blunted amygdala reactivity to interpersonal threat and might even be an important confounder in the widely documented association between childhood maltreatment and threat-related amygdala response, which needs to be further investigated in future longitudinal studies. Differences in sample characteristics (for example comorbidities), experimental designs (the use of highly threatening pictures versus resting-state or individual recall of stressful situations), and analysis techniques (focusing only on dissociation or controlling for modulating factors) may explain part of the discrepancies in previous studies. More research is needed to better understand how precisely dissociative symptoms may lead to the proposed dampening of amygdala activity and whether this is restricted to certain subgroups or high levels of pathological dissociation.

6.3 Psychophysiological Research

In their systematic review, Roydeva and Reinders [70] included psychophysiological studies that measured electrodermal activity (skin conductance response, SCR), heart rate, heart rate variability, blood pressure, and startle responses. None of these measures was consistently associated with pathological dissociation across disorders. Another recent systematic review focused exclusively on psychophysiological responses to traumatic material (including 28 eligible studies, with overall $N =$ 1.300 participants [214]. There was again no clear trend or pattern since some studies found a decrease in heart rate and a blunting of autonomic arousal, while others found hyperactive autonomic responses to traumatic content. There was tentative evidence for a closer association between acute dissociative states or self-reported peritraumatic dissociation with autonomic hypo-reactivity. In some studies in patients with a primary BPD diagnosis, acute dissociation was associated with reduced startle responses [364, 365], diminished skin conductance response to aversive stimuli [271] and increased high-frequency heart rate variability (indicating higher parasympathetic activity over sympathetic activity) during an instructed emotion regulation task [366]. Comorbidity with PTSD in these samples was relatively high. In another study in adolescents with BPD, dissociation was positively correlated with relative heart rate habituation to acoustic startle probes (sinus tones), suggesting an influence on automatic defensive responses [367]. In line with this, another study in adult BPD patients found a moderating effect of dissociative symptoms on psychophysiological responses, including SCR [368]. While these findings indicate a modulating role of dissociation on autonomic arousal in BPD, contradictory findings were also reported, see [70, 214].

Overall, empirical evidence for a blunting of autonomic arousal as a potential physiological marker of dissociation is mixed [70]. As mentioned before, possible reasons for the lack of robust findings are the high diversity of study groups, assessments of dissociation, and psychophysiological parameters, among other methodological aspects [70, 214]. Adaptation times, measurement durations, and baseline conditions were different, which could have contributed to inconsistencies [214]. This again underscores the complexity of investigating dissociation, also in a laboratory setting, and shows the challenges in identifying consistent psychophysiological correlates, calling for a multi-methodological assessment of dissociation [214].

Importantly, a recent study investigated associations between dissociative symptoms and behavioural, physiological, and experiential threat responses in individuals with PTSD [342]. Using the aforementioned script-driven imagery paradigm, participants underwent either a standardized script, a detail-enriched trauma script, or a neutral script. Stabilometry, eye-tracking, facial electromyography, autonomic psychophysiology, and self-reports were assessed. In addition, PTSD symptoms were assessed before and 3 months after testing. While the analyses did not show a link between acute dissociation and bodily, facial immobility or staring in response to trauma scripts, an inverted U-shaped relationship with psychophysiological measures was detected. Patients showed higher non-specific skin conductance fluctuation and higher high-frequency heart rate variability in response to trauma scripts. Acute dissociation was linked to higher self-reported negative affect responses to trauma scripts and displayed a U-shaped relationship with unfavorable PTSD symptom course. With respect to these psychophysiological markers of dissociation, results support the defence cascade model of an inverted U-shaped relationship between dissociation and psychophysiological arousal. Increases in dissociation may be associated with a progressive increase of parasympathetic over sympathetic activation. These non-linear associations may help explain the heterogeneity and inconsistency of prior findings [342].

Overall, there is evidence that alterations in dorsomedial and dorsolateral prefrontal cortical brain areas, bilateral superior frontal regions, (anterior) cingulate, posterior association areas, and basal ganglia may be transdiagnostic neural markers of pathological dissociation, independent of the primary psychiatric diagnosis [70]. For BPD specifically, increased activity in the inferior frontal gyrus and inferior, middle, and superior temporal gyrus as well as decreased activity in temporo-occipital regions (fusiform gyrus, cuneus, lingual gyrus), posterior cingulate, precuneus, and amygdala were found [10]. All in all, this suggests that dissociation may be associated with alterations in brain networks implicated in emotion processing, cognitive control and arousal modulation, self-referential processing, interoception, body representation, and the filtering, processing, and integration of sensory input. As emphasized before, findings are still quite diverse and cover a wide range of clusters in the brain, and could not always be replicated.

In general, neurobiological research on pathological dissociation is still in its infancy and the precise neurobiological underpinnings remain elusive. Studies used different operationalizations and measures of dissociation [360], which hinders a straightforward interpretation and comparison of studies. State and trait dissociation may have different or even opposite neurobiological correlates and only few studies so far investigated the impact of acute dissociation, for example, using script-driven imagery or pharmacological agents [16, 28, 273, 362]. Studies need sufficient and robust statistical power to have the potential to detect possible biomarkers. Moreover, recent research highlights the need to use ultra-high field imaging to gain a more sensitive picture of the neural connectivity underlying psychopathology [369].

CHAPTER 7

Implications for BPD

Abstract In BPD, dissociative experiences are highly common, but also very diverse in their manifestations and severity. Acute dissociative symptoms typically occur during emotional stress, often together with psychotic or psychotic-like symptoms. Chronic dissociative symptoms are often intertwined with other BPD features, such as reduced emotional awareness, identity disturbances, and self-harming behaviour. Therefore, dissociation may be either overlooked or considered a mere consequence of distress. However, research suggests that dissociation is not merely a learned stress response or maladaptive coping mechanism, but also a predisposition to more serious problems in emotion regulation, identity disturbances, and interpersonal conflict. When assessed in daily life, dissociation was not only triggered by stress, but also worsened affective instability and relationship problems. Dissociation appears to be more severe and persistent in individuals with adverse childhood experiences, long-lasting trauma, and co-occurring mental health conditions. Neurobiological and experimental studies suggest that dissociative states are associated with a hyposensitivity to pain and social threat, possibly due to dampened autonomic arousal and limbic reactivity, as well as impaired emotional learning and memory. Findings underline the need to understand dissociative symptoms in a broader biosocial framework and to carefully evaluate their individual manifestations, functions, and possible impact on everyday life and treatment.

A. Krause-Utz, *Dissociation in Borderline Personality Disorder*, https://doi.org/10.1007/978-3-032-06339-7_7

Keywords Borderline personality disorder · Emotion dysregulation · Identity diffusion · Interpersonal disturbances · Stress

The complex, multifaceted nature of dissociation calls for a more nuanced understanding of dissociative symptoms in BPD. Acute dissociative states under stress are considered a hallmark feature of the disorder [14, 15]. However, manifestations of dissociation can be very diverse, and some individuals with BPD do not only experience transient dissociative states but also chronic dissociation, such as profound depersonalization, self-alienation, identity confusion, and memory fragmentations. Dissociative experiences appear to be more severe and persistent in patients with more severe symptoms, functional impairments, and hospital admissions, partly due to comorbid disorders, such as PTSD and dissociative disorders [7, 9]. In BPD, the presence of other debilitating symptoms can easily overshadow dissociative symptoms if they are not clearly expressed and carefully examined. When dissociation is accompanied by emotional dysregulation, self-harm, and psychotic episodes, it may be overlooked or considered secondary. However, chronic dissociation can be a risk factor for a more severe and chronic course of the disorder if it is not addressed as a relevant treatment target [20–22].

Empirical findings provide support for prominent theories of BPD that proposed how dissociative symptoms are related to reduced stress tolerance, problems in emotion regulation [113, 370], mentalization problems [236, 237], disturbed internal representations of self and others [223], and maladaptive schemas and schema modes [301, 371]. The biosocial theory by Linehan [464] proposes that highly sensitive children with low distress tolerance and unstable emotions can develop a pattern of profound emotional dysregulation if they grow up in an invalidation environment, in which the "communication of private experiences is met by erratic, inappropriate, and extreme response" by primary caregivers (Linehan [464, p. 42]).

The highly sensitive temperament, lack of other coping resources, and unsupportive, invalidating social environment increase the risk of dissociation in individuals with BPD. Similar to people with recognized neurodivergent conditions such as autism and ADHD, people with BPD may "shut-down" in overwhelming situations, because they are easily overwhelmed by emotions, thoughts, sensations, and social demands.

Dissociation can protect against emotional and sensory overload, which may lead people with BPD to consciously or unconsciously use it as a maladaptive coping strategy. While dissociation can provide temporary relief, it can increase affective instability in the long term.

Mentalization-based theories of BPD highlight the role of attachment disruptions that impair the ability to understand one's own and others' mental states and result in mentalization deficits [240]. Dissociation has not only been associated with early life stress and attachment-related stressors (see Sect. 4.1.3.3) but also with reduced emotional and bodily awareness. Being out of touch with one′s emotions, bodily sensations, needs, and personal experiences can be alienating, leading to both profound self-alienation and difficulties with intimacy in close relationships [236].

Schema theory highlights the role of early maladaptive schemas related to adverse childhood experiences in the way how individuals with BPD perceive themselves, others, and the world around them [371]. Schemas of defectiveness and shame, vulnerability to harm, and social isolation can go hand in hand with dissociative experiences and both may mutually reinforce each other [305]. Frequent dissociative experiences may reinforce negative self-beliefs of being helpless, powerless, unloved, and isolated. If the potentially self-perpetuating nature of dissociation is not understood, people may blame themselves for not taking action and staying in a detached protector mode, which helps to cut off emotional pain, shame, and guilt but also leads to social isolation and feelings of alienation and loneliness [304, 309]. The perpetuating nature of schemas may increase the risk of a vicious cycle where dissociative experiences and core beliefs influence the way current events are perceived [37, 308]; see Sect. 4.5.

All in all, dissociative symptoms are best understood in the context of other BPD symptoms. As illustrated in Fig. 7.1, all of these symptoms and their complex interplay should be understood in a biosocial context. Together with other core features of the disorder, such as emotional dysregulation, identity disturbance, and interpersonal problems, dissociation may present an ongoing challenge that should be examined and targeted in a person-centred manner. Empirical evidence for this interplay is addressed below for each symptom domain.

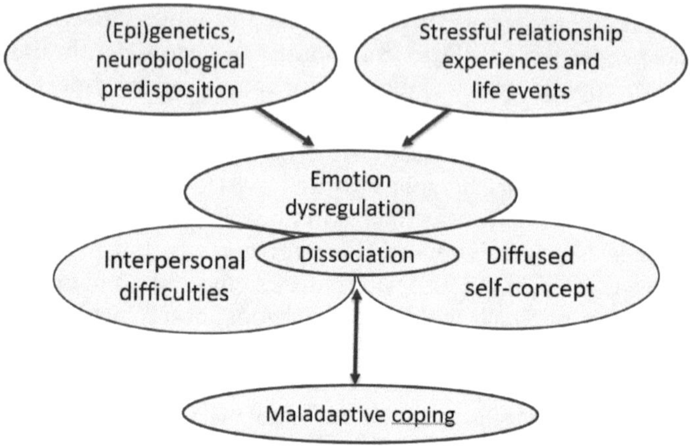

Fig. 7.1 The biosocial model of borderline personality disorder

7.1 Emotion Dysregulation and Stress Reactivity

Emotion regulation is considered a core feature of BPD, associated with heightened emotional sensitivity, intense, unstable emotions, and the use of maladaptive emotion regulation strategies [372–374]. Dissociative experiences, such as depersonalization and derealization, are more common in people who tend to suppress or avoid difficult emotions [296]. Individuals with chronic dissociative experiences often have limited awareness of their needs, impulses, or physical sensations, and more problems detecting early warning signs or triggers for emotional distress. This diminished ability to identify and express emotions or bodily states has been associated with more somatic expressions of distress [8, 31, 106, 298, 299]. In BPD, dissociative experiences may worsen preexisting emotion regulation difficulties.

Emotional distress, in turn, is a common trigger for dissociative states [1, 15, 182, 312, 313, 315]. Increases in dissociative symptoms followed subjective increases in affective arousal [312]. Individuals with BPD often have reduced stress tolerance, which can make them more vulnerable to various types of stressors and more prone to become overwhelmed in emotionally challenging situations. Dissociation may be an unconscious automatically triggered stress response, while some people may actively induce dissociation to protect themselves from overwhelming emotions, sensations, and pain.

In one study [314], dissociation also predicted subsequent affective fluctuations, which highlights that dissociation is not only a consequence but also a risk factor for higher distress and emotional instability in BPD. A possible reason for this may be that dissociative experience reactivate maladaptive schemas related to shame, defectiveness, and isolation [305]. Moreover, dissociation may interfere with problem solving and lead to more interpersonal conflicts, which are a potent trigger for emotional distress in BPD.

7.2 Repetitive Self-Harm and Altered Body Perceptions

Non-suicidal self-injury can be one of many maladaptive coping strategies that individuals with BPD use to regulate stress and to deal with interpersonal conflicts. Compared to healthy people, individuals with BPD usually experience lower pain sensitivity and their pain thresholds are even higher during stress-related states of dissociation [28, 318]. Stress-related pain analgesia has been linked to a stronger urge to self-harm in BPD, which may have various reasons [27]. On the one hand, dissociation may lower the inhibition threshold for non-suicidal self-injury because it is less painful then. On the other hand, research suggests that some people purposely use self-injury in a manner that intentionally induces pain [375]. In an anonymous online survey, completed by a large sample ($N = 1.630$) from the general population who reported self-harm histories, higher levels of dissociation were associated with less subjective pain during self-injury. The offset of pain was associated with reductions in emotional pain. However, participants more often reported an onset than an offset of pain related to self-injury. In that respect, findings suggest that people may not only use self-harm to reduce pain, but also in a manner that induces pain [375].

Another common motive for self-harm is to terminate unwanted dissociative states that provoke anxiety and cause distress [27, 318, 321, 376]. There is growing evidence for altered body perception in people with BPD who frequently experience dissociation [24, 25, 322]. In this case, self-harm may be used to regain a sense of control and agency, to end states of emotional and physical numbness [236, 321, 377, 378]. Self-harm, such as cutting or burning, might then be maladaptive attempts to manage strong and uncontrollable dissociation. This again highlights the need to evaluate the presence of dissociative symptoms in individuals BPD.

7.3 Unstable Identity and Self-Image

Identity disturbance is another core feature of BPD. Individuals with the disorder do not only have the subjective experience of a markedly unstable, vague or fragmented sense of self; they also show objective incoherencies in thought, feeling, and behaviour [379]. Strongly fluctuating self-images [380] and the accuracy of self-reflections are influenced by rapid changes in affect [381, 382]. Pre-existing problems in goal-setting and future planning could be worsened by dissociation, which can make it harder to understand and explain own needs and motives and identify consistent goals and values [8, 379]. The reactivation of early maladaptive schemas and schema modes related to self-blame, shame, guilt, and self-loathing may partly underlie extreme changes in mood, self-image, and behaviours, reminiscent of DID [301, 303]. At the same time, it should be highlighted that identity disturbances in BPD are not only related to negative beliefs (of being abandoned, worthless, unlovable, incompetent, and helpless), but also associated with alterations in socio-cognitive and self-referential processing [379, 382, 383].

7.4 Interpersonal Disturbances

Interpersonal disturbances are the third core domain of BPD symptoms. Individuals with BPD are usually highly sensitive to social threat and rejection while experiencing profound loneliness and a strong need to belong [383–385]. They often exhibit ambivalent attachment styles, partly due to adverse childhood experiences and insecure attachment relationships with primary caregivers [386]. A lack of social problem-solving skills and assertiveness can lead to difficulties in setting healthy boundaries and expressing own needs in interpersonal situations. Some people with BPD show impulsive anger and aggression when stressed or frustrated, which is another source for interpersonal conflicts [387–389].

For some individuals with BPD, dissociation may be a learned maladaptive strategy for coping with interpersonal conflict. In the short term, dissociation may help to distance oneself from hostile confrontations and to escape painful feelings of rejection but also intense anger and aggression. At the same time, dissociation may lead to anger, incomprehension, and rejection in others, prolonging interpersonal conflicts. Unwantedly, this can lead to a collapse of important relationships, a reinforcement of old patterns [386], and both a reactivation and confirmation of early maladaptive schemas [310]. As previously mentioned, interpersonal conflicts were found to be important triggers for dissociation when assessing symptoms over time in everyday life [314]. Moreover, there is evidence that dissociation increases the risk of revictimization [245, 249, 250], possibly due to reduced risk perception and impulsive risk-taking [30], particularly in individuals with difficulties in emotion regulation and impulsivity—two core features of BPD [317, 390, 391].

7.5 Environmental Influences and the Role of Interpersonal Stress and Trauma

It is important to consider various etiological pathways in the development of both BPD and chronic dissociation. It is currently assumed that BPD develops from a complex interplay of genetic, neurobiological vulnerability and environmental stressors, including both trauma-related and non-trauma related pathways [112]. Similarly, dissociative disorders usually develop from an interplay of dispositions and stressors; see Sect. 4.

While not all individuals with BPD experience dissociation and dissociation in BPD is not always linked to trauma, numerous studies suggest that dissociative experiences are more prevalent and more persistent in groups with adverse childhood experiences and severe trauma histories, possibly due to comorbidities, such as PTSD and CPTSD [12, 126, 136, 137]. Rates of childhood abuse and neglect are substantially higher in BPD compared to other psychiatric groups, including depression and other personality disorders [146, 392]. There is evidence that emotional forms of abuse and neglect are particularly relevant to BPD [146, 393]. Harsh or insensitive parenting [146, 392], disorganized attachment interactions with a parent [394, 395], and bullying victimisation during adolescence [238, 396] were associated with the development and symptom severity of BPD. Adverse childhood experiences can hinder the development of emotion regulation, self-control, and identity, and contribute to problems in self-regulation at later developmental stages [220, 221]. Abuse and neglect can have long-lasting effects on brain development and neurobiological processes [218, 219] and such changes can also occur due to other stressful interpersonal experiences, for example parental unavailability [224]. The development of dissociative tendencies may then be understood as part of an ongoing psychological and neurobiological adaptation to aversive environments [106–108, 197].

Several studies in groups with BPD found associations between dissociative experiences and adverse childhood experiences as well as repeated trauma in adolescence and adulthood [136, 198, 397]. Using semi-structured interviews to assess adverse childhood experiences and interpersonal violence in adulthood, one study found that inconsistent treatment by a caretaker, sexual abuse by a caretaker, witnessing sexual violence as a child, and adult rape history predicted levels of dissociation in BPD [198]. Findings from prospective studies suggest that dissociative experiences are not only more prevalent in groups with higher psychopathological load and trauma histories but also more persistent over time [126, 136, 137]. Severity of childhood sexual abuse, adult history of rape, and adult history of partner violence predicted higher levels of trait dissociation (DES scores) over the course of 24 years in individuals with a BPD diagnosis and individuals with other personality disorders [137]. However, other studies found no associations between dissociation and childhood trauma and the presence of co-occurring disorders, such as PTSD, might explain some discrepancies [302]. Therefore, it is important to consider a possible history of trauma in individuals with BPD who report severe levels of dissociation, while carefully avoiding a one-sided approach and a suggestive questioning style. A too narrow focus on trauma does not adequately account for the complexity of dissociation and might even cause iatrogenic harm.

Scientifically, more research is needed to understand if the onset, timing, and source of trauma plays a role in the development and maintenance of dissociation in BPD in comparison with clinical control groups [141, 392]. The impact of stressful life experiences and trauma on the development of dissociative symptoms in BPD should also be understood from a broader biopsychosocial perspective that considers modulating factors and mediating mechanisms [193]. Poor sleep, physical exhaustion, substance use, and sensory overload may be influencing vulnerability factors [37, 38, 192, 193, 285], see Sect. 4. Individuals with mental disorders and trauma histories often find it difficult to sufficiently care for themselves, have intrusive nightmares and use dissociation-inducing substances to self-medicate and numb emotions. These can be triggers for acute dissociative episodes [37, 38, 192, 193, 285].

7.6 Neurobiology

Neurobiological genetic predispositions play a role in the development of BPD. There is evidence for a highly heritable factor (55%) in BPD [398], although no single genetic factor has been associated with BPD and there is genetic overlap with bipolar disorder, major depression, and schizophrenia [399]. Some studies found alterations in the hypothalamic–pituitary–adrenal (HPA) axis and serotonergic system, although contradictory findings of increased versus decreased cortisol levels were also found [400, 401]. Alterations in the endogenous opioid system may be involved in self-harming behaviours in BPD [402].

Neurobiological studies revealed functional and structural alterations in brain regions implicated in emotional and social-cognitive processing, such as the amygdala, hippocampus, insula, anterior cingulate, orbitofrontal cortex, and medial prefrontal cortex [403–407]. Dissociation has been associated with altered structure and activity in these brain circuitries (see Sect. 6.2). Because dissociative symptoms usually co-occur with other BPD symptoms, it is difficult to disentangle their neurobiological underpinnings. However, the finding of dampened amygdala activity and increased prefrontal control is of importance here, since individuals with BPD typically exhibit amygdala hyperreactivity. A comprehensive meta-analysis showed that amygdala hyperreactivity to threatening stimuli is more pronounced in BPD patients than in depressed samples, which may underlie increased emotional sensitivity and intense and prolonged emotional reactions [408]. Individuals with BPD showed diminished habituation to repeated negative stimuli, which was associated with adverse childhood experiences [409].

During acute dissociation, individuals with BPD showed reduced amygdala reactivity to threatening images [16, 334, 410] and dampened amygdala-modulated autonomic arousal [365, 368]. These findings could underlie the diminished emotional reactivity and experiential detachment from threat during stress-related dissociative episodes in BPD. While a dampening of arousal is useful and adaptive during acute inescapable threat, it can become counterproductive in situations where there is no current threat, as it can impair habituation to feared stimuli [365, 368, 410]. While more research is needed to replicate these findings in larger groups with BPD, a recent study in a large samples of individuals with adverse childhood experiences found strong evidence that dissociation is associated with blunted bilateral amygdala reactivity to interpersonal threat and might even be an important confounder in the widely documented association between childhood maltreatment and amygdala hyperreactivity [358]. More research is needed if a reduction in dissociative symptoms leads to a normalization of amygdala reactivity. While amygdala reactivity to negative versus neutral images predicted poor individual treatment response to dialectical behaviour therapy [411], the successful treatment of emotion regulation led to a normalization or lower levels of amygdala reactivity to threat [403, 406, 412, 413]. Research suggests that brain activation patterns can change after treatment [414]. Treatment responders demonstrated reduced activation in amygdala, anterior cingulate cortex, orbitofrontal, and dorsolateral prefrontal cortex together with increased connectivity within a limbic-prefrontal network during the reappraisal of negative stimuli after psychotherapy [415]. A reduction of amygdala activity to relatively normal levels could also be achieved through real-time fMRI neurofeedback training of amygdala hemodynamic activity aimed at a conscious downregulation of own amygdala blood oxygen-level-dependent responses [416]. It still needs to be investigated how this is linked to the frequency of dissociation.

Earlier neurobiological findings suggested that diminished prefrontal control underlies clinically observed problems in emotion regulation and impulse control in BPD, see [407]. However, this earlier assumption was challenged due to methodological problems, such as a lack of spatial and disease specificity [373]. Diminished activity in dorsolateral and orbitofrontal regions has not consistently been replicated [373] and may be restricted to subgroups with anger-related aggression [387, 417]. At the same time, several neuroimaging studies in BPD have consistently found increased activity in the inferior frontal gyrus [16, 273, 376] and other frontal areas. Alterations in dorsomedial and dorsolateral prefrontal cortical brain areas, bilateral superior frontal regions, (anterior) cingulate, and posterior association areas, were found across groups with dissociative symptoms and may point to increased efforts of cognitive control or emotion modulation [70, 357].

Increased activation in temporal areas (inferior, middle, and superior temporal gyrus) and decreased activity in temporo-occipital regions (fusiform gyrus, cuneus, lingual gyrus), posterior cingulate, and precuneus, and the amygdala were also found in groups with BPD [10]. All in all, these finding point to alterations in brain areas implicated in sensory processing, self-referential processing, and memory. At the same time, findings are still diverse and need to be replicated. Conceptual differences and methodological differences in the assessment of dissociation hinder a straightforward interpretation and comparison of studies.

While the neurobiological underpinnings of dissociation are not yet fully understood, experimental neuroimaging research suggests that acute dissociation can interfere with affective-cognitive processing, including emotional learning and memory in BPD. On the neural level, this may be associated with alterations in cortico-limbic and temporal regions (including the amygdala, hippocampus, insula, anterior cingulate, orbitofrontal cortex, and medial prefrontal cortex) that might also underlie other BPD symptoms, such as emotion dysregulation, impulsivity, and identity disturbance [403, 404, 407].

7.7 Suggestions for Future Studies and Qualitative Research

Integrating self-reports, experimental tasks, neuroimaging assessments, and clinical interventions could help to better understand whether changes in dissociation are accompanied by changes in neurocognitive performance and a normalization of brain activity. This could also help to identify subgroups that may benefit most from certain interventions aimed at reducing dissociative psychopathology.

More research is needed to understand whether specific dissociative symptoms have a differential impact on information processing and psychopathological outcomes in BPD. There is tentative evidence that depersonalization and derealization may be closely connected to affective instability and identity disturbances, while dissociative amnesia may be connected to self-harming impulsivity [33]. However, these hypotheses need to be tested in homogenous clinical samples. Future studies could investigate if and how acute dissociative states influence the processing of emotional expressions and trustworthiness in unfamiliar faces or other social cues, while controlling for general alterations in social cognition (mentalizing, empathy, theory of mind). Since earlier studies found that these aspects of social cognition were altered in BPD, they should be considered as possible confounders [418–420].

Most studies so far focused on the impact of dissociation on the processing of negative material. However, growing evidence suggests that people with BPD also show an altered perception of positive social signals—including pleasant touch, positive social feedback, or smile—and have difficulties detecting and memorizing positive social events, possibly due to a negativity bias [323, 382, 421–425]. Individuals with BPD seem to engage less in social interactions that could enhance feelings of happiness and joy [335]. A reduced ability to experience or enhance positive emotions could be related to chronic dissociation, which may lead to a more fragmented sense of self and exacerbate identity problems. However, this association still needs to be investigated and better understood. Most experimental studies so far used highly aversive or threatening stimuli to investigate the impact of dissociation on emotional processing and regulation. Whether dissociation interferes with the processing and memory of positive information still needs to be investigated.

Moreover, more qualitative research in the field is needed to understand how dissociation manifests itself in everyday life situations. Narratives of individuals with lived experiences could give insight into how dissociative states affect important life domains. An unpublished thematic analysis of autobiographical dissociation scripts collected in a group of women with a primary BPD diagnosis and severe childhood trauma [16, 17] was conducted to gain some preliminary insights into the content of these scripts (in preparation/unpublished data by the author). It was explored whether qualitatively distinct forms of dissociation could be identified in these autobiographical narratives and whether they were are associated with overarching themes (recurrent and prevalent topics).

Results of this exploratory thematic analysis indicated qualitatively distinct forms of dissociation, which largely correspond to the experiences of detachment (for example, *"I notice how reality starts to feel further away"*; *"it seems like a film that is passing me by"*; *"everything is blurred/strange/blurry"*, *"people around me look like ants"*). Some excerpts explicitly described physical and emotional numbing (*"I don't have to feel my feelings anymore"*), out of body experiences (*"I step out of my body"*), self-induced absorption (*"I fixate on a point on the wall and notice how I slowly drift away*; *"I keep rocking back and forth and fixate my eyes onto the corridor [until] I no longer notice anything else"*, *"I stare out of the window"*), disruptions in attention and memory (*"my memory fails me"*, *"my brain shuts down"*, *"I can hear myself from far away"*; *"the questions I am asked do not reach me."*; *"I hear the words of the others, but I don't understand them, they flow through me"*), or difficulties speaking and moving (“*I can't move anymore*”, “*I cannot feel my legs, my body*”, “*I collapse*”).

Four overarching themes were identified: interpersonal conflicts (volatile family dynamics, fights, aggressive arguments, rejection by a friend, coworker, or partner, but also witnessing other peoples′ struggles and suffering), strong negative emotions (feeling tense, stressed, and overwhelmed, afraid, panicking, angry, powerless, isolated, and embarrassed), physical stress reactions (consistent with sympathetic nervous system activation or acute stress responses, such as heart racing, shortness of breath, difficulty breathing), and perceived threat with the explicit wish to escape. Interpersonal situations described in the scripts involved various social contacts (friends, family, romantic partner, therapist, fellow patients, co-workers, or fellow student) and also mentioned being overwhelmed by witnessing the suffering of others. Interpersonal or threatening situations and negative emotions preceded dissociative experiences, while physical reactions co-occurred with dissociative experiences. These very first preliminary findings need to be followed up using more extensive qualitative interviews in representative samples. A combination of qualitative and quantitative research and a more careful assessment of dissociative phenomena and potentially confounding variables, such as trauma history, will help to further increase the understanding of underlying mechanisms and functions.

Ideally, future studies should include multiple measures, such as a combination of neuroimaging, psychophysiological, interviews, and self-report, as well as different qualitative and quantitative analytical techniques, and also include clinical control groups. Shared etiologies, especially trauma histories, should be taken into account [8, 10, 31]. To better understand the potential role of trauma, future studies should include groups of participants who experienced trauma without developing psychiatric disorders. Distinguishing between state and trait dissociation and using repeated measure designs or ambulatory assessment methods can help to better understand whether observed alterations are relatively stable or associated with transient states.

Findings from studies described so far suggest that emotion dysregulation (including affective instability and maladaptive coping), negative self-image (including early maladaptive schemas), potentially self-harming impulsivity, and adverse interpersonal experiences may all be correlated to more severe dissociative experiences. These features are not only associated with a diagnosis of BPD, but can also occur in other clinical groups and, to lower extents, in the general population. Dimensional models conceptualize personality disorders, such as BPD, as a pattern of traits (persistent ways of thinking, feeling, and behaving) that are maladaptive extremes of traits that are normally distributed in the general population [132, 133, 426]. From this point of view, associations between dissociative symptoms and BPD features (affective instability, impulsivity, identity diffusion, negative relationship experiences) do not need to be limited to groups of people who meet criteria for a personality disorder diagnosis.

7.8 Methodological Challenges and Limitations

Given the wide spectrum of dissociative symptoms, different studies might have captured different aspects of dissociation in different subgroups, which may explain some of the discrepancies and a lack of consistent findings. While dissociation is a transdiagnostic phenomenon, a direct comparison of studies can be difficult given the potential influence of sample characteristics (gender, trauma histories, comorbidities, medication status, etc.), measures, designs, and analysis techniques. Among others, most studies included women. Although dissociative disorders are more frequently diagnosed in women than in men, both biological sexes are affected equally and the diversity in biological sex and gender needs to be taken into account [79]. The co-occurrence of BPD, dissociative disorders, and PTSD is highly representative for clinical groups with high levels of dissociation. At the same time, the presence of comorbidities may have confounded some results. To this date, the number of studies with clinical comparison groups is too low to draw firm conclusions with regard to disorder-specific or transdiagnostic effects.

Findings from correlational studies that used self-reports face several methodological limitations, as the observed correlations might have been influenced (confounded, moderated, or mediated) by other factors, not investigated in the study. Self-reports generally include the risk of over- and underreporting symptoms, for example due to conscious or unconscious recall biases, such as a lack of insight, shame, or socially desired responses. Correlational observational studies which use retrospective self-reports cannot establish temporal causality. Longitudinal, prospective studies are needed to better understand whether dissociation precedes, coincides with, or follows certain observations or alterations and to determine causal temporal relationships.

In general, rigor inclusion and exclusion criteria increase the quality of well-defined groups with respect to specific diagnoses but this hampers recruitment and often results in small sample sizes. Studies with larger sample sizes with sufficient statistical power are needed to extend and replicate previous findings [357]. Larger meta-analysis can help to compare effect sizes from various studies and identify possible moderators and mediators. These methodological challenges and limitations prevent a clear interpretation of findings. For a thorough interpretation, the interested reader should take a closer look at the study´s conceptualization, operationalization, and assessment of dissociation and the study population.

CHAPTER 8

Treatment

Abstract Psychotherapy is considered the first choice and gold standard in the treatment of dissociative disorders. At the moment, different treatment options are available. For complex dissociative disorders, guidelines of the International Society for the Study of Trauma and Dissociation recommend a phase-oriented staged approach, which is integrative, flexible, and preferably long-term. Modifications of personality disorder treatments and trauma-focused treatments have also been found to effectively treat individuals with severe dissociation. Several modified protocols are currently tested. For BPD, clinical staging models are recommended instead of a one-fits-all approach. Treatment guidelines for BPD recommend that co-occurring disorders, such as dissociative disorders, should be managed concurrently with BPD-specific treatment and should only be prioritized if the co-occurring disorder prevents effective psychotherapy or leads to a life-threatening situation. There is evidence that dissociative symptoms can be effectively targeted with established or modified versions of specialized treatments for BPD, such as dialectical behaviour therapy, mentalization-based treatment, transference-focused therapy, and schema therapy. Dissociative symptoms should be carefully assessed at different stages of the therapeutic process. Depending on the individual triggers and functions of dissociation, different practical skills and personalized interventions can be used to counteract dissociative symptoms within and outside of therapy sessions.

A. Krause-Utz, *Dissociation in Borderline Personality Disorder*,
https://doi.org/10.1007/978-3-032-06339-7_8

Keywords Interventions · Psychotherapy · Therapy · Treatment · Protocols

Psychotherapy is regarded as the first choice and gold standard in the treatment of dissociative disorders [12, 169]. Across different schools, dissociation is viewed as a complex construct, which warrants a thorough assessment of symptoms, including differential diagnosis before the start of psychotherapy [12, 169]. In general, dissociation should be carefully screened at different stages of the therapeutic process and personalized interventions should be utilized to optimize treatment. Psychoeducation about dissociation, dissociative disorders, attachment, emotion regulation, traumatization, and survival strategies should be standard parts of the treatment [169]. A comprehensive case formulation should consider the biopsychosocial diatheses (genetic, neurobiological predispositions, risk factors, protective factors), previous and current stressors, including trauma and other stressful life events, as well as currently maintaining factors. Realistic personal treatment goals should be formulated through joint decision-making and a crisis or emergency plan should be established. Several treatment forms and modified protocols were found to decrease symptoms of dissociation. Experts recommend a flexible approach, which may alternate between stages of stabilization and trauma-informed interventions, depending on the current state of symptoms, daily functioning, emotion regulation, and quality of life [428].

8.1 Phase-Oriented Approach

For complex dissociative disorders, guidelines of the International Society for the Study of Trauma and Dissociation (ISSTD) recommend a phase-oriented staged approach, which is integrative, flexible, and preferably long term [169]. The phase-oriented approach is based on the assumption that early interpersonal trauma, including abuse and/or neglect, plays an important role in the development of chronic dissociation and disorders, such as DID, and that the long duration of dissociative experiences is accompanied by profound difficulties in stress regulation and identity. The phase-oriented treatment starts with stabilization, followed by trauma processing. Clients first learn how to manage their dissociative symptoms, regulate strong emotions, and develop or improve interpersonal skills. This first phase aims to create safety and stability by building a strong, trusting, and supportive therapeutic relationship, and promoting skills needed to cope with everyday life that can later be used for trauma processing. This skills training is combined with psychoeducation. When the client is ready and stable enough, the next step is taken aimed at working through stressful past experiences and trauma by using techniques such as EMDR, imaginary exposure, narrative exposure therapy (NET), and cognitive restructuring, focusing on trauma-related core beliefs and feelings such as guilt and shame. For DID, the long-term goal is a guided integration of the personality parts or a better internal cooperation between them. Attention is paid to grief, relapse prevention, finding new values, and future planning. There is evidence that clients report fewer dissociative and PTSD symptoms, less depression, less drug use, fewer physical pain complaints, and less dangerous and self-injurious behaviour and suicide attempts with progressing treatment phases, see [168, 169]. For groups with other mental disorders who experience dissociation, including PTSD and BPD, other treatment approaches recommend to immediately start with trauma processing, as long as it is complemented with psychoeducation, skills training, and a close monitoring of dissociative symptoms before, during, and after exposure, see for example [429, 430].

8.2 Trauma-Focused Treatments

Trauma-focused treatment recommend by the National Institute for Health and Care Excellence (NICE) guidelines are Cognitive Behavioral Therapy (TF-CBT), Cognitive Processing Therapy (CPT), Prolonged Exposure (PE), and Eye Movement Desensitization and Reprocessing (EMDR) as first-line treatments for PTSD [272]. Meta-analyses showed that EMDR and TF-CBT are effective in reducing PTSD symptoms and improving remission rates in adults with PTSD [431, 432].

Trauma-focused cognitive behavioural therapy involves cognitive restructuring, psychoeducation, and emotion regulation skills training in addition to the repeated exposure to traumatic memories [433]. During imaginary exposure or in-vivo exposure, clients are repeatedly confronted with distressing memories and experiences or real-life situations (objects, smells, and people) that are related to the traumatic experience but are inherently harmless. The assumed working mechanism of prolonged exposure is that repeated exposure to feared stimuli facilitates emotional processing and habituation, leading to a decrease in stress reactions. By activating the fear network, feared expectations are challenged. Through repeated practice, clients learn how to confront and integrate traumatic memories while discovering that these memories and trauma-related stimuli are not harmful. The therapist provides a safe space and support, while ensuring that the client does not avoid trauma-related emotions, feelings, thoughts, and physical sensations, or use avoidance strategies. It is assumed that dissociative responses will diminish simultaneously with other avoidance responses after successful trauma processing, when they are no longer necessary. With the help of the practitioner, the client also learns how to recognize and stop dissociation, and to tolerate strong emotions. Ultimately, this process is expected to result in a decrease in PTSD symptoms [434].

In EMDR, traumatic processing is facilitated by recalling the traumatic experience while simultaneously incorporating bilateral stimulation, such as eye movements, taps, or sounds. The dual attention task is hypothesized to be the underlying mechanism of EMDR, taxing working memory and limiting attentional resources to maintain the vividness of traumatic memories; this is thought to lead to less emotionally charged memories and thus a reduction of PTSD symptoms [435]. EMDR includes relatively little verbal instruction, as the client is not explicitly encouraged to verbalize the trauma memories.

8.3 Modified Personality Disorder Treatments

There is evidence that modifications of personality disorder treatments are effective in dissociative disorders, such as DID. Dialectical behaviour therapy (DBT), mentalization-based treatment (MBT), transference-focused therapy (TFT), and schema-focused therapy (SFT) are established personality disorder treatments, for example for the treatment of BPD [436], which were modified for dissociative and trauma-related disorders, as briefly introduced below.

8.3.1 Dialectical Behaviour Therapy (DBT)

Standard DBT is a combination of individual therapy, group therapies (skills training), team meetings, and constant supervision in a multi-disciplinary setting. In a dialectical synthesis, acceptance and validation is combined with change-oriented strategies, aimed at the acquisition of practical skills and pragmatic problem-solving. A trustful and strong therapeutic relationship is established, fostered by a deepened understanding of the origin and individual expressions of problems. At the same time, practical skills in the areas of mindfulness (living fully in the present moment), distress tolerance, emotion regulation, and interpersonal effectiveness skills are taught. While working towards recovery, small progressive steps are promoted and relapses are anticipated, using techniques of motivational interviewing and validation.

A modified form of DBT for dissociative disorders has been developed [437] and is currently being tested in its effectiveness for individuals with dissociative disorders. Other modified protocols were developed for individuals with complex trauma [429, 430], see below. It is assumed that teaching skills in stress tolerance, emotion regulation, and mindfulness can help to reduce the frequency of dissociation [296, 438]. Depending on the individual's triggers and functions of dissociation, different skills can be used to counteract dissociation in DBT [438]. It often takes time to find the most effective skill per person. If dissociation primarily functions as a coping mechanism to escape or numb overwhelming emotions in stressful situations, DBT self-soothing techniques and distress tolerance skills, such as the use of ice packs, a stress ball, or strong scents, can be used to reduce unwanted dissociative symptoms [438, 439]. As described above, acute dissociation is often triggered by extreme stress levels, which are more common in BPD [113, 370]. In addition, DBT emotion regulation skills can help the client to better identify, understand, and tolerate difficult emotions. Radical acceptance can help to overcome past painful experiences that cannot be changed anymore in order to focus on the present and to build a life that is worth living. Interpersonal effectiveness skills can be implemented to develop more stability in social interactions and to deal with interpersonal conflicts that are known triggers for dissociation. Grounding, breathing, and mindfulness techniques can help anchor the client in the present and promote an increased awareness of bodily sensations, emotions, and thoughts. Learning to observe and describe one's internal and external experiences without judgment can help to reduce the automatic response of dissociation [279, 440, 441]. Especially in clients with trauma histories, re-engaging with bodily sensations often involves discomfort or even traumatic re-experiencing, which needs to be prepared and discussed. In general, it is crucial to acknowledge, validate, and anticipate the ambivalences many people experience when asked to let go of dissociation. Since dissociation often served as a survival mechanisms, the pros and cons need to be discussed in an open and validating way [236].

8.3.2 *Modified DBT Protocols for PTSD*

Modified protocols of DBT were developed for individuals with BPD and comorbid PTSD related to childhood abuse. The first protocol by Harned et al. [430, 442] combines DBT with Prolonged Exposure (PE) therapy (DBT + PE) and was evaluated in different studies [430, 442]. It is a staged approach that starts with a stabilization phase to establish therapeutic commitment, a safe and trustful relationship, and treatment goals. The aim of this first phase is to reduce high-risk behaviours. Clients gain more control over self-damaging impulsive behaviours. It is ensured that they fully committed to subsequent trauma treatment and have sufficient behavioural control or skills to manage intense distress during trauma-focused therapy. This protocol was found to be effective in reducing the severity of PTSD symptoms [430, 442]. Reductions in dissociation were found along with decreases in self-harm, suicide attempts, and trauma-related guilt, anxiety, shame, and depression [430, 442].

Bohus et al. [443, 444] developed a protocol for individuals with BPD symptoms and PTSD after interpersonal trauma (sexual and physical abuse in childhood), called DBT-PTSD. This adaptation combines DBT with trauma-focused interventions (Cognitive Therapy and prolonged exposure) and elements of Acceptance and Commitment Therapy [445] and Compassion Focused Therapy (CFT) [446]. It can be offered both as inpatient and outpatient treatment settings. It has a clear focus on dealing with dissociation within sessions, especially during exposure. In DBT-PTSD, trauma exposure starts earlier in the process but is assisted with simultaneous skills training. Clients learn how to apply their skills during difficult therapy sessions and also learn to be more compassionate with themselves, more forgiving, and more mindful. A first randomized-control trial (RCT) comparing a 12-week residential DBT-PTSD treatment to a treatment-as-usual wait list showed a significantly greater change in PTSD symptoms without an increase in dysfunctional behaviours for DBT-PTSD [444]. In a second large multicentre RCT, DBT-PTSD was tested against Cognitive Processing Therapy (CPT) over the course of a year and three follow-up months [443]. Significantly, fewer women dropped out prematurely from DBT-PTSD (39%

vs. 25.5%). Both CPT and BPD-PTSD resulted in a reduction of PTSD symptoms, with a slightly greater and more reliable change in DBT-PTSD. Only DBT-PTSD resulted in a reduction of dissociative symptoms, BPD symptoms, and depression, and the DBT-PTSD group had higher remission rates (40.7% vs. 58.4%). Findings support the efficacy of DBT-PTSD and CPT for treating women with childhood abuse-associated complex PTSD and provide preliminary evidence for a slight superiority of DBT-PTSD.

In DBT-PTSD much emphasis is paid on the use of anti-dissociation skills, especially during exposure to internal or external cues that symbolize or resemble the traumatic event(s). During skills-assisted exposure, anti-dissociation skills, such as balancing boards, are used to counteract dissociation within the therapy session to improve the ability to learn new associations and unlearn old associations [429].

Research suggests that dissociation may interfere with core principle of trauma-focused treatments, including the integration of memories in a personal narrative and the learning of new associations (see Sect. 4. 1.3.5). While the effect of dissociation on PTSD treatment is controversial [270], baseline dissociation was a negative predictor for treatment efficacy of DBT-PTSD in individuals with PTSD related to childhood abuse [20, 22]. These findings suggest that high levels of dissociation can prevent trauma-focused psychological therapies from reaching their full potential. This does not argue against including highly dissociative individuals into treatments. Instead, it highlights the need of monitoring and targeting these symptoms carefully. The disruptive role of dissociation during psychotherapy might be particularly pronounced in individuals, who enter treatment with high levels of symptom severity, and it is conceivable that dissociation particularly affects treatment progress in this group [21]. Besides common strategies of teaching skills, mindfulness, and reducing vulnerabilities, the implementation of anti-dissociative strategies as part of trauma-focused psychotherapy seems to be needed.

8.3.3 Mentalization-Based Therapy (MBT)

With MBT, clients learn to better understand and explain their motives and the motives of others by "mentalizing" needs and beliefs that underlie certain behaviours [236, 238, 240]. In a collaborative trustful relationship, client and therapist investigate situations in which mentalization decreases and discuss how this leads to specific symptoms and problems in daily life and therapy sessions. As previously mentioned, dissociation is assumed to be one of many factors that can reduce mentalization abilities, often due to adverse childhood experiences and difficult attachments with primary caregivers [236, 238]. An important aim of MBT is to foster epistemic trust, both in the therapeutic relationship and with respect to trusting own experiences. This process involves authenticity, transparency, and clarification of misunderstandings and intentions, including the admission of errors and readiness to repair therapeutic relationship ruptures, while encouraging the client to develop a sense of agency and control [240, 427]. A modified version of MBT has been developed for people with complex trauma, which explicitly targets dissociative symptoms [236, 237]. The underlying assumption is that generalized improvements in overall mentalizing capacity can be achieved by fostering a reflective process with regard to traumatic experiences and dissociative symptoms. This staged approach that on stabilization and psychoeducation before the processing of traumatic memories, followed by a phase in which mourning, acceptance of loss, and moving on are central. It can be implemented over a period of 6 months as an adjunct to standard MBT, or over 9–12 months as a stand-alone intervention [236, 237]. Interventions typically begin by clearly identifying the dissociative state, assessing the client′s present needs to soothe or ground them and guiding the patient to self-regulate. Within a group setting, a safe space is offered to reflect on the dissociative experience and to mentalize it later [236]. More effectiveness studies for this modification, including randomized-controlled trials, for this modification are still needed.

8.3.4 *Transference-Focused Therapy (TFT)*

Transference-focused psychotherapy (TFP) is another evidence-based treatment for BPD [127, 447], which has been used to treat dissociative disorders. Dissociation is considered a defence mechanism, which leads to disturbed representations of others and oneself [223]. The distorted perceptions of self and others are the focus of the treatment. It is assumed that common and central interpersonal and emotional problems will also reveal themselves in the relationship with the therapist. The therapeutic relationship is therefore central. For DID, the treatment aim is to integrate disconnected parts and to achieve a more consistent interpretation of distorted perceptions. Case studies describe the application of TFT to the treatment of DID [448], while effectiveness studies, including randomized-controlled trials are still needed.

8.3.5 Schema-Focused Therapy (SFT)

Schema therapy combines cognitive behavioural, interpersonal, and experiential techniques and was found to be effective in treating personality disorders, such as BPD [436, 449]. It has been modified for treating dissociative disorders, including DID [450, 451]. Schema theory argues that abrupt shifts in emotion, cognition, and behaviour, which can be seen in BPD and DID, can largely be explained by a reactivation of different underlying schemas and schema modes [301, 371]. Changes in behaviour and emotions are seen as manifestations of recurring, rigid schema modes. Switching between different schema modes can be accompanied by a strong sense of discontinuity in emotional experience and self-image. Two case studies describe a reduction in complex dissociative symptoms with schema therapy [450, 451]. Modified schema therapy for DID includes a strong emphasis on experiential techniques. Metaphors are used to help the client understand and validate basic needs, feelings, thoughts, and behaviour. Traumatic experiences are processed through imaginary rescripting. This integrated approach aims to allow the patient to meet the basic needs of the child modes and to achieve more consciousness and control over dysfunctional modes [452]. Schema therapy has not yet been established for patients with complex dissociative disorders, but empirical evaluations of the applicability of schema therapy for DID are currently ongoing [452].

8.3.6 Unified protocol (UP)

The unified protocol (UP) assumes that complex disorders, such as personality disorders and dissociative disorder, are associated with a core deficit in self-regulation and disturbed emotion regulation [453–455]. Strategies that promote cognitive, emotional, and behavioural regulation are assumed to lead to a reduction in dissociative symptoms. If traumatic memories are involved, the UP focuses on the processing and regulation of associated negative emotions, such as shame, and their role in the perception of trauma (for example, through cognitive restructuring). Similar to trauma-focused treatments, the UP mostly views dissociative symptoms as an avoidance of such emotions. The UP has been shown to be effective in several RCTs in the treatment of anxiety, depression, and BPD, but still needs to be more explicitly studied in patients with DID and other complex dissociative disorders.

8.4 Implications for BPD Treatment

Psychotherapy is the main treatment for BPD [456] and several specialized and evidence-based treatments, including DBT, MBT, TFT and SFT, exist [436]. Instead of a one-fits-all approach,

clinical staging models are recommended, depending on clinical severity [457, 458], especially since specialist treatments are resource-intensive and limited [457, 459–461]. Individuals with less pronounced BPD symptoms may benefit from psychoeducation, problem-solving skills training, and elements of effective specialist treatments provided by non-PD-specialist mental health professionals [460, 462]. Individuals with severe and persistent BPD symptoms who are heavily impaired in their psychosocial functioning and show pathology that requires specialist psychosocial treatment need to be referred to specialized intensive treatment [458].

Treatment guidelines for BPD recommend that co-occurring disorders, such as dissociative disorders, should be managed concurrently with BPD-specific treatment and should only be prioritized if the co-occurring disorder prevents effective psychotherapy or leads to a life-threatening situation [463]. Even if BPD is the primary diagnosis, however, dissociative symptoms should be carefully assessed and targeted before, during, and after treatment. As described above, there is evidence that dissociative symptoms can be effectively targeted with established specialized treatments for BPD, such as DBT [464], MBT [240, 465], TFP [466], and ST [301, 371] although randomized-control trials for some of the modified protocols are still needed or currently underway.

Common therapeutic strategies to tackle dissociative symptoms in BPD include a comprehensive case conceptualization, psychoeducation, personalized treatment goals, and balancing a patient empathic validating approach with practical skills training. As already emphasized, the careful assessment of dissociative symptoms is essential to fully understand and capture the manifold individual expressions of dissociative symptoms. Since dissociation manifest itself very differently, a comprehensive case formulation should consider different biopsychosocial influences, developmental trajectories, and previous and current stressors. While severe dissociative symptoms appear to be more common in BPD patients with complex trauma histories [198], suggestive questioning should be avoided [169] and multiple risk factors other than trauma should be considered as well. Dissociative symptoms can generalize to situations that are highly stressful but only indirectly related to past stressful events [467]. Besides stress-related symptoms of detachment, the full range of symptoms should be considered, including dissociative absorption, symptoms of compartmentalization, and somatoform manifestations [6, 468]. Coming up with such a case formulation can take some time. An inherent aspect of dissociation is the disconnection from internal and external experiences [438]. Oftentimes, clients first need to learn how to observe, monitor, and label their dissociative experiences in connection with emotions, thoughts, and physiological sensations and how they are connected to external triggers. Warning signs across different situations first need to be established. Psychoeducation about dissociation can help clients to become more aware of typical triggers and symptoms and should therefore be a standard part of treatment [169]. Depending on the individual triggers and functions of dissociation, different practical skills (for example, from DBT [438, 439] or mindfulness-based interventions [279, 440, 441] can be used to counteract these symptoms. Guided by the therapist, clients can learn to identify the events or chain of events that lead to severe dissociative episodes, including dissociative flashbacks [236, 438]. Improving sleep quality and regular fluid intake can also help to reduce the vulnerability to experience dissociation.

Overall Summary and Conclusion

Dissociation is a multifaceted transdiagnostic phenomenon that refers to disruptions of normally integrated mental functions. The severity of dissociative experiences varies widely, ranging from non-pathological forms of dissociation to severe dissociative disorders. Manifestations of pathological dissociation include symptoms of detachment (depersonalization and derealization) and compartmentalization, up to severe fragmentation of emotions, through, identity, and memory. The etiology of dissociative disorders usually involves an interplay of various factors, including neurobiological temperamental dispositions, psychological stress, trauma, socio-cognitive, and cultural factors.

Dissociation is highly common in BPD. Yet, the severity, intensity, and duration of dissociative symptoms vary considerably. The most prominent manifestation of dissociation in BPD is an acute breakdown of mental functions during intense emotional distress, often accompanied by severe emotion dysregulation, psychotic symptoms, self-harm, or suicidal behaviour. However, dissociation in BPD should not be merely viewed as a stress reaction or avoidance mechanism. In some people with BPD, chronic experience of dissociation may have evolved from a interplay of genetic neurobiological dispositions and various influences beyond stress and trauma. In some cases, dissociative symptoms may be more subtle and masked by other debilitating symptoms, co-occurring mental and physical health problems, and comorbidities such as PTSD and CPTSD. It is highly important to detect this subgroup of individuals who may not only

A. Krause-Utz, *Dissociation in Borderline Personality Disorder*,
https://doi.org/10.1007/978-3-032-06339-7

have greater problems in emotion regulation, self-damaging, risk-taking behaviours, and a more negative self-image, but also struggle with chronic dissociation.

If left unaddressed, symptoms, such as difficulties in emotion regulation, reduced stress tolerance, identity alterations, and interpersonal sensitivity, and dissociation may reinforce each other, contributing to a vicious cycle that maintains the disorder. Research findings reviewed in this pivot showed that dissociative experiences are closely associated with reduced stress tolerance, distorted body perception, emotional and interpersonal sensitivity, impulsivity, and altered pain processing. These associations are likely reciprocal. Momentary assessments in everyday life show that dissociation is not only a maladaptive stress response, but can also lead to increased affective instability and interpersonal conflict, possibly due to secondary emotions of guilt, helplessness, and shame. Furthermore, acute dissociation can dampen fear responses and impair emotional learning and memory. This not only represents an important risk factor for (re)victimization in violent abuse situations but also has important implications for treatment. It also suggests that addressing other emotion dysregulation, mentalization problems, dysfunctional schemas, and interpersonal problems may help to reduce dissociation and vice versa [113, 371, 427].

Given the manifold manifestations of dissociation, it is important to examine them more closely and understand how personal experiences have shaped their development and maintenance. Distinguishing between acute dissociative states and general tendencies, as well as specific types of dissociative experiences can be helpful in this regard. Not all forms of dissociation are necessarily pathological, and a person-centred empathic and validating approach can help to carefully understand the adaptive and maladaptive aspects of dissociative experiences. A trusting relationship, psychoeducation about the negative consequences of dissociation, and training in anti-dissociation skills can help those affected to control dissociation and to let go of this protective strategy in moments where it is harmful and maladaptive. Once alternative strategies are learned and support is provided, dissociation may become less or at least more manageable.

Acute dissociation may interfere with treatment processes aimed at an integration of autobiographical memories, emotional experiences, habituation to feared stimuli, and cognitive restructuring. Importantly, this does not mean that patients with severe dissociation should be excluded from such treatments or that this group benefits less from these approaches overall. Instead, it highlights the need to make dissociation an important aspect of treatment, understanding its nature and impact and potential ways it could interfere with treatment and daily life in general. Patients should learn how to strengthen their stress tolerance and emotion regulation skills, their social support systems, and their interpersonal effectiveness. Addressing maladaptive schemas and past traumatic life experiences can also reduce vulnerability and help people with chronic dissociative experiences to reconnect with their lives.

References

1. American Psychiatric Association. Diagnostic and statistical manual of mental disorders [Internet]. DSM-5-TR. American Psychiatric Association Publishing; 2022 [cited 2024 July 15]. Available from: https://doi.org/10.1176/appi.books.9780890425787
2. Spiegel D, Lewis-Fernández R, Lanius R, Vermetten E, Simeon D, Friedman M. Dissociative disorders in DSM-5. Annu Rev Clin Psychol. 2013;9(1):299–326.
3. Brown RJ. Different types of "dissociation" have different psychological mechanisms. J Trauma Dissociation. 2006;7(4):7–28.
4. Spiegel D, Cardeña E. Disintegrated experience: the dissociative disorders revisited. J Abnorm Psychol. 1991;100(3):366–78.
5. Waller N, Putnam FW, Carlson EB. Types of dissociation and dissociative types: a taxometric analysis of dissociative experiences. Psychol Methods. 1996;1(3):300–21.
6. Lyssenko L, Schmahl C, Bockhacker L, Vonderlin R, Bohus M, Kleindienst N. Dissociation in psychiatric disorders: a meta-analysis of studies using the dissociative experiences scale. AJP. 2018;175(1):37–46.
7. Salavati M, Selby EA. Dissociation in borderline personality disorder. In: Theories of borderline personality disorder [Internet]. Cham: Springer Nature Switzerland; 2024 [cited 2025 Jan 28]. p. 225–45. Available from: https://doi.org/10.1007/978-3-031-75503-3_10
8. Brand BL, Lanius RA. Chronic complex dissociative disorders and borderline personality disorder: disorders of emotion dysregulation? Bord Personal Disord Emot Dysregul. 2014;1(1):13.

A. Krause-Utz, *Dissociation in Borderline Personality Disorder*, https://doi.org/10.1007/978-3-032-06339-7

9. Al-Shamali HF, Winkler O, Talarico F, Greenshaw AJ, Forner C, Zhang Y, et al. A systematic scoping review of dissociation in borderline personality disorder and implications for research and clinical practice: exploring the fog. Aust N Z J Psychiatry. 2022;56(10):1252–64.
10. Krause-Utz A, Frost R, Chatzaki E, Winter D, Schmahl C, Elzinga BM. Dissociation in borderline personality disorder: recent experimental, neurobiological studies, and implications for future research and treatment. Curr Psychiatry Rep. 2021;23(6):37.
11. Scalabrini A, Cavicchioli M, Fossati A, Maffei C. The extent of dissociation in borderline personality disorder: a meta-analytic review. J Trauma Dissociation. 2017;18(4):522–43.
12. Brand BL. The concise guide to the assessment and treatment of trauma-related dissociation. [Internet]. Washington: American Psychological Association; 2024 [cited 2025 Feb 21]. Available from: https://content.apa.org/books/17343-000
13. Korzekwa MI, Dell PF. Is dissociation an integral aspect of borderline personality disorder, or is it a comorbid disorder? In M. J. Dorahy, S. N. Gold, & J. A. O'Neil (Eds.), Dissociation and the dissociative disorders: Past, present, future. In: 2nd ed. Routledge; 2023. p. 494–512.
14. American Psychiatric Association. Diagnostic and Statistical Manual of Mental Disorders, Fifth edition. 2013.
15. WHO. International Classification of Diseases 11th Revision [Internet]. World Health Organization; 2019. Available from: https://icd.who.int/en
16. Krause-Utz A, Winter D, Schriner F, Chiu CD, Lis S, Spinhoven P, et al. Reduced amygdala reactivity and impaired working memory during dissociation in borderline personality disorder. Eur Arch Psychiatry Clin Neurosci. 2018;268(4):401–15.
17. Winter D, Krause-Utz A, Lis S, Chiu CD, Lanius RA, Schriner F, et al. Dissociation in borderline personality disorder: disturbed cognitive and emotional inhibition and its neural correlates. Psychiatry Res Neuroimaging. 2015;233(3):339–51.
18. Ebner-Priemer UW, Mauchnik J, Kleindienst N, Schmahl C, Peper M, Rosenthal MZ, et al. Emotional learning during dissociative states in borderline personality disorder. J Psychiatry Neurosci. 2009;34(3):214–22.
19. McKinnon MC, Boyd JE, Frewen PA, Lanius UF, Jetly R, Richardson JD, et al. A review of the relation between dissociation, memory, executive functioning and social cognition in military members and civilians with neuropsychiatric conditions. Neuropsychologia. 2016;90:210–34.
20. Kleindienst N, Priebe K, Görg N, Dyer A, Steil R, Lyssenko L, et al. State dissociation moderates response to dialectical behavior therapy for posttraumatic stress disorder in women with and without borderline personality disorder. Eur J Psychotraumatol. 2016;7(1):30375.

21. Kleindienst N, Steil R, Priebe K, Müller-Engelmann M, Lindauer P, Krause-Utz A, et al. Is dissociation predicting the efficacy of psychological therapies for PTSD? Results from a randomized controlled trial comparing Dialectical Behavior Therapy for PTSD (DBT-PTSD) and Cognitive Processing Therapy (CPT). Psychol Med. 2025;55: e59.
22. Kleindienst N, Limberger MF, Ebner-Priemer UW, Keibel-Mauchnik J, Dyer A, Berger M, et al. Dissociation predicts poor response to dialectial behavioral therapy in female patients with borderline personality disorder. J Pers Disord. 2011;25(4):432–47.
23. Wedig MM, Silverman MH, Frankenburg FR, Reich DB, Fitzmaurice G, Zanarini MC. Predictors of suicide attempts in patients with borderline personality disorder over 16 years of prospective follow-up. Psychol Med. 2012;42(11):2395–404.
24. Bekrater-Bodmann R, Chung BY, Foell J, Gescher DM, Bohus M, Flor H. Body plasticity in borderline personality disorder: a link to dissociation. Compr Psychiatry. 2016;69:36–44.
25. Löffler A, Kleindienst N, Cackowski S, Schmidinger I, Bekrater-Bodmann R. Reductions in whole-body ownership in borderline personality disorder—a phenomenological manifestation of dissociation. J Trauma Dissociation. 2020;21(2):264–77.
26. Chung BY, Hensel S, Schmidinger I, Bekrater-Bodmann R, Flor H. Dissociation proneness and pain hyposensitivity in current and remitted borderline personality disorder. Eur J Pain. 2020;24(7):1257–68.
27. Bohus M, Limberger M, Ebner U, Glocker FX, Schwarz B, Wernz M, et al. Pain perception during self-reported distress and calmness in patients with borderline personality disorder and self-mutilating behavior. Psychiatry Res. 2000;95(3):251–60.
28. Ludäscher P, Valerius G, Stiglmayr C, Mauchnik J, Lanius RA, Bohus M, et al. Pain sensitivity and neural processing during dissociative states in patients with borderline personality disorder with and without comorbid posttraumatic stress disorder: a pilot study. J Psychiatry Neurosci. 2010;35(3):177–84.
29. Van Schie C, Gallagher R, Krause-Utz A. Exploring the complex relationship between childhood trauma and self-harm. J Aggress Maltreat Trauma. 2024;2024:1–19.
30. Mazinan RG, Dudek C, Warkentin H, Finkenstaedt M, Schröder J, Musil R, et al. Borderline personality disorder and sexuality: causes and consequences of dissociative symptoms. Bord Personal Disord Emot Dysregul. 2024;11(1):8.
31. Ford JD, Courtois CA. Complex PTSD and borderline personality disorder. Bord Personal Disord Emot Dysregul. 2021;8(1):16.
32. Bach B, Kramer U, Doering S, Di Giacomo E, Hutsebaut J, Kaera A, et al. The ICD-11 classification of personality disorders: a European perspective on challenges and opportunities. Bord Personal Disord Emot Dysregul.

2022;9(1):12.
33. Schulze A, Hughes N, Lis S, Krause-Utz A. Dissociative experiences, borderline personality disorder features, and childhood trauma: generating hypotheses from data-driven network analysis in an international sample. J Trauma Dissociation. 2024;2024:1–20.
34. Fung HW, Wong MYC, Lam SKK, Wong ENM, Chien WT, Hung SL, et al. Borderline personality disorder features and their relationship with trauma and dissociation in a sample of community health service users. Borderline Personal Disord Emot Dysregul. 2023;10(1):22.
35. Fayad M, Scheer V, Blanco C, Louville P, Sánchez-Rico M, Rezaei K, et al. Identifying bridge symptoms between borderline personality disorder and posttraumatic stress disorder: a network analysis from a national cohort. J Clin Psychiatry. 2024;85(4):23m15079.
36. Knefel M, Tran US, Lueger-Schuster B. The association of posttraumatic stress disorder, complex posttraumatic stress disorder, and borderline personality disorder from a network analytical perspective. J Anxiety Disord. 2016;43:70–8.
37. Lynn SJ, Polizzi C, Merckelbach H, Chiu CD, Maxwell R, Van Heugten D, et al. Dissociation and dissociative disorders reconsidered: beyond sociocognitive and trauma models toward a transtheoretical framework. Annu Rev Clin Psychol. 2022;18(1):259–89.
38. Sar V, Krüger C, Martínez-Taboas A, Middleton W, Dorahy M. Sociocognitive and posttraumatic models of dissociation are not opposed. J Nervous Ment Dis. 2013;201(5):439–40.
39. Cardeña E. The domain of dissociation. In: Lynn SJ, Rhue JW, editors. Dissociation: clinical and theoretical aspects. New York: Guilford Press; 1994. p. 5–31.
40. Şar V. The many faces of dissociation: opportunities for innovative research in psychiatry. Clin Psychopharmacol Neurosci. 2014;12(3):171–9.
41. Briere J, Weathers FW, Runtz M. Is dissociation a multidimensional construct? Data from the Multiscale Dissociation Inventory. J Traum Stress. 2005;18(3):221–31.
42. Dell PF. The multidimensional inventory of dissociation (MID): a comprehensive measure of pathological dissociation. J Trauma Dissociation. 2006;7(2):77–106.
43. Fung HW, Chau AKC, Lam SKK, Chien WT, Wong JYH. A cross-cultural study of different facets of dissociation: Validity and relationship with childhood trauma. Child Abuse Negl. 2024;157: 107067.
44. Şar V. Dissociation across cultures: a transdiagnostic guide for clinical assessment and management. Alpha Psychiatry. 2022;23(3):95–103.
45. Spitzer C, Barnow S, Freyberger HJ, Grabe HJ. Recent developments in the theory of dissociation. World Psychiatry. 2006;5(2):82–6.

46. Van der Hart O, Nijenhuis E. Dissociative disorders. Oxford: Oxford University Press; 2009.
47. Cardeña E, Carlson E. Acute stress disorder revisited. Annu Rev Clin Psychol. 2011;7(1):245–67.
48. Dell PF, O'Neil JA. Dissociation and the dissociative disorders: DSM-V and Beyond. New York, NY US: Routledge/Taylor & Francis Group; 2009.
49. Soffer-Dudek N, Lassri D, Soffer-Dudek N, Shahar G. Dissociative absorption: an empirically unique, clinically relevant, dissociative factor. Conscious Cogn. 2015;36:338–51.
50. Soffer-Dudek N. Dissociative absorption, mind-wandering, and attention-deficit symptoms: associations with obsessive-compulsive symptoms. Br J Clinic Psychol. 2019;58(1):51–69.
51. Waller NG, Ross CA. The prevalence and biometric structure of pathological dissociation in the general population: Taxometric and behavior genetic findings. J Abnorm Psychol. 1997;106(4):499–510.
52. Butler LD. Normative dissociation. Psychiatr Clin North Am. 2006;29(1):45–62.
53. Waller N, Putnam FW, Carlson EB. Types of dissociation and dissociative types: a taxometric analysis of dissociative experiences. Psychol Methods. 1996;1(3):300–21.
54. Janet P. The mental state of hystericals: a study of mental stigmata and mental accidents. London: GP Putnam's Sons; 1901.
55. Holmes E, Brown R, Mansell W, Fearon R, Hunter E, Frasquilho F, et al. Are there two qualitatively distinct forms of dissociation? A review and some clinical implications. Clin Psychol Rev. 2005;25(1):1–23.
56. Veltman DJ, De Ruiter MB, Rombouts SARB, Lazeron RHC, Barkhof F, Van Dyck R, et al. Neurophysiological correlates of increased verbal working memory in high-dissociative participants: a functional MRI study. Psychol Med. 2005;35(2):175–85.
57. De Ruiter MB, Phaf RH, Veltman DJ, Kok A, Van Dyck R. Attention as a characteristic of nonclinical dissociation: an event-related potential study. Neuroimage. 2003;19(2):376–90.
58. Thomson P, Jaque SV. History of childhood adversity and coping strategies: positive flow and creative experiences. Child Abuse Negl. 2019;90:185–92.
59. Dalenberg CJ, Brand BL, Gleaves DH, Dorahy MJ, Loewenstein RJ, Cardeña E, et al. Evaluation of the evidence for the trauma and fantasy models of dissociation. Psychol Bull. 2012;138(3):550–88.
60. Schauer M, Elbert T. Dissociation following traumatic stress: etiology and treatment. Z Psychol J Psychol. 2010;218(2):109–27.
61. Kozlowska K, Walker P, McLean L, Carrive P. Fear and the defense cascade: clinical implications and management. Harv Rev Psychiatry. 2015;23(4):263–87.

62. Putnam FW. Diagnosis and treatment of multiple personality disorder. 2. [print.]. New York: Guilford Pr; 1989. 351 p. (Foundations of modern psychiatry).
63. Spiegel D, Cardeña E. Disintegrated experience: the dissociative disorders revisited. J Abnorm Psychol. 1991;100(3):366–78.
64. Sar V. Epidemiology of dissociative disorders: an overview. Epidemiol Res Int. 2011;2011:1–8.
65. Şar V. Dissociative depression is resistant to treatment-as-usual. JPCPY [Internet]. 2015 July 30 [cited 2025 May 18];3(2). Available from: https://medcraveonline.com/JPCPY/dissociative-depression-is-resistant-to-treatment-as-usual.html
66. Sar V, Akyüz G, Öztürk E, Alioğlu F. Dissociative depression among women in the community. J Trauma Dissociation. 2013;14(4):423–38.
67. Parish A, Reuben K. Dissociation in autism spectrum disorders: an under-recognized symptom. In: Perspectives of dissociative identity response: ethical, historical, and cultural issues; 2022.
68. Bozkurt H, Duzman Mutluer T, Kose C, Zoroglu S. High psychiatric comorbidity in adolescents with dissociative disorders. Psychiatry Clin Neurosci. 2015;69(6):369–74.
69. Sebastian A, Jung P, Krause-Utz A, Lieb K, Schmahl C, Tüscher O. Frontal dysfunctions of impulse control—a systematic review in borderline personality disorder and attention-deficit/hyperactivity disorder. Front Hum Neurosci. 2014;8:698.
70. Roydeva MI, Reinders AATS. Biomarkers of pathological dissociation: a systematic review. Neurosci Biobehav Rev. 2020;S0149763420306485.
71. North C. The classification of hysteria and related disorders: historical and phenomenological considerations. Behav Sci. 2015;5(4):496–517.
72. Hart O, Horst R. The dissociation theory of Pierre Janet. J Trauma Stress. 1989;2(4):397–412.
73. Foote B, Smolin Y, Kaplan M, Legatt ME, Lipschitz D. Prevalence of dissociative disorders in psychiatric outpatients. AJP. 2006;163(4):623–9.
74. Kate MA, Hopwood T, Jamieson G. The prevalence of dissociative disorders and dissociative experiences in college populations: a meta-analysis of 98 studies. J Trauma Dissociation. 2020;21(1):16–61.
75. Friedl MC, Draijer N, de Jonge P. Prevalence of dissociative disorders in psychiatric in-patients: the impact of study characteristics. Acta Psychiatr Scand. 2000;102(6):423–8.
76. Kedare JS, Baliga SP, Kadiani AM. Clinical practice guidelines for assessment and management of dissociative disorders presenting as psychiatric emergencies. Indian J Psychiatry. 2023;65(2):186–95.

77. Ross CA, Duffy CMM, Ellason JW. Prevalence, reliability and validity of dissociative disorders in an inpatient setting. J Trauma Dissociation. 2002;3(1):7–17.
78. Sar V, Koyuncu A, Ozturk E, Yargic LI, Kundakci T, Yazici A, et al. Dissociative disorders in the psychiatric emergency ward. Gen Hosp Psychiatry. 2007;29(1):45–50.
79. Spitzer C, Freyberger HJ. Geschlechtsunterschiede bei dissoziativen Störungen. Bundesgesundheitsbl. 2008;51(1):46–52.
80. Krüger C. Culture, trauma and dissociation: a broadening perspective for our field. J Trauma Dissociation. 2020;21(1):1–13.
81. Fung HW, Ling HWH, Ross CA, Tse JWL, Liu RKW. Dissociative, Schneiderian and borderline personality symptoms in a non-clinical sample in Hong Kong: a preliminary report. Eur J Trauma Dissociation. 2020;4(1): 100076.
82. Chiu CD, Tseng MCM, Chien YL, Liao SC, Liu CM, Yeh YY, et al. Switch function and pathological dissociation in acute psychiatric inpatients. PLoS ONE. 2016;11(4): e0154667.
83. Chiu CD, Ho HL, Tollenaar MS. Relational self-evaluations in dissociation: Implicit self-rejection? Psychol Trauma. 2022;14(1):99–106.
84. Fung HW, Chan C, Chien WT, Chong YY, Ross CA. The acceptability and potential benefits of a web-based psychoeducation program for people with pathological dissociation: a pilot evaluation study. J Trauma Dissociation. 2023;24(1):95–110.
85. Xiao Z, Yan H, Wang Z, Zou Z, Xu MDY, Chen MDJ, et al. Trauma and dissociation in China. AJP. 2006;163(8):1388–91.
86. Brand BL, Sar V, Stavropoulos P, Krüger C, Korzekwa M, Martínez-Taboas A, et al. Separating fact from fiction: an empirical examination of six myths about dissociative identity disorder. Harv Rev Psychiatry. 2016;24(4):257–70.
87. Bhavsar V, Ventriglio A, Bhugra D. Dissociative trance and spirit possession: challenges for cultures in transition. Psychiatry Clin Neurosci. 2016;70(12):551–9.
88. Bhugra D, Bhui K, editors. Textbook of cultural psychiatry [Internet]. 1st ed. Cambridge University Press; 2007 [cited 2024 July 14]. Available from: https://www.cambridge.org/core/product/identifier/9780511543609/type/book
89. Staniloiu A, Markowitsch HJ. Dissociative amnesia. Lancet Psychiatry. 2014;1(3):226–41.
90. American Psychiatric Association. Diagnostic and statistical manual of mental disorders : DSM-5. fifth edition. Arlington, VA; 2013.
91. Reinders AATS, Marquand AF, Schlumpf YR, Chalavi S, Vissia EM, Nijenhuis ERS, et al. Aiding the diagnosis of dissociative identity disorder: pattern recognition study of brain biomarkers. Br J Psychiatry. 2019;215(3):536–44.

92. Koenen KC, Ratanatharathorn A, Ng L, McLaughlin KA, Bromet EJ, Stein DJ, et al. Posttraumatic stress disorder in the World Mental Health Surveys. Psychol Med. 2017;47(13):2260–74.
93. Møller L, Augsburger M, Elklit A, Søgaard U, Simonsen E. Traumatic experiences, ICD-11 PTSD, ICD-11 complex PTSD, and the overlap with ICD-10 diagnoses. Acta Psychiatr Scand. 2020;141(5):421–31.
94. Wolf EJ, Mitchell KS, Sadeh N, Hein C, Fuhrman I, Pietrzak RH, et al. The dissociative subtype of PTSD scale: initial evaluation in a national sample of trauma-exposed veterans. Assessment. 2017;24(4):503–16.
95. Hansen M, Ross J, Armour C. Evidence of the dissociative PTSD subtype: a systematic literature review of latent class and profile analytic studies of PTSD. J Affect Disord. 2017;213:59–69.
96. Hyland P, Shevlin M, Fyvie C, Cloitre M, Karatzias T. The relationship between ICD-11 PTSD, complex PTSD and dissociative experiences. J Trauma Dissociation. 2020;21(1):62–72.
97. Hyland P, Karatzias T, Shevlin M, Cloitre M, Ben-Ezra M. A longitudinal study of ICD-11 PTSD and complex PTSD in the general population of Israel. Psychiatry Res. 2020;286: 112871.
98. Fung HW, Yuan GF, Liu C, Lin ESS, Lam SKK, Wong JYH. Prevalence and clinical correlates of dissociative symptoms in people with complex PTSD: Is complex PTSD a dissociative disorder? Psychiatry Res. 2024;339: 116076.
99. Hyland P, Hamer R, Fox R, Vallières F, Karatzias T, Shevlin M, et al. Is dissociation a fundamental component of ICD-11 complex posttraumatic stress disorder? J Trauma Dissociation. 2024;25(1):45–61.
100. Jowett S, Karatzias T, Shevlin M, Hyland P. Psychological trauma at different developmental stages and ICD-11 CPTSD: the role of dissociation. J Trauma Dissociation. 2022;23(1):52–67.
101. Herman J. Trauma and recovery: the aftermath of violence—from domestic abuse to political terror. New York, NY US: Basic Books; 1992.
102. Brewin CR, Cloitre M, Hyland P, Shevlin M, Maercker A, Bryant RA, et al. A review of current evidence regarding the ICD-11 proposals for diagnosing PTSD and complex PTSD. Clin Psychol Rev. 2017;58:1–15.
103. Hyland P, Karatzias T, Shevlin M, McElroy E, Ben-Ezra M, Cloitre M, et al. Does requiring trauma exposure affect rates of ICD-11 PTSD and complex PTSD? Implications for DSM–5. Psychol Trauma Theory Res Pract Policy. 2021;13(2):133–41.
104. van der Kolk BA. Developmental trauma disorder: towards a rational diagnosis for chronically traumatized children. Prax Kinderpsychol Kinderpsychiatr. 2009;58(8):572–86.
105. Maercker A. Development of the new CPTSD diagnosis for ICD-11. Borderline Personal Disord Emot Dysregul. 2021;8(1):7.

106. Ford JD, Spinazzola J, Van Der Kolk B, Grasso DJ. Toward an Empirically Based Developmental Trauma Disorder Diagnosis for Children: Factor Structure, Item Characteristics, Reliability, and Validity of the Developmental Trauma Disorder Semi-Structured Interview. J Clin Psychiatry [Internet]. 2018 Sept 11 [cited 2024 Aug 18];79(5). Available from: https://www.psychiatrist.com/jcp/developmental-trauma-disorder-advancing-toward-an-empirically-based-diagnosis
107. Schimmenti A, Caretti V. Linking the overwhelming with the unbearable: developmental trauma, dissociation, and the disconnected self. Psychoanal Psychol. 2016;33(1):106–28.
108. D'Andrea W, Ford J, Stolbach B, Spinazzola J, Van Der Kolk BA. Understanding interpersonal trauma in children: why we need a developmentally appropriate trauma diagnosis. Am J Orthopsychiatry. 2012;82(2):187–200.
109. Ross CA, Ridgway J, George N. Maladaptive daydreaming, dissociation, and the dissociative disorders. Psychiatr res clin pract. 2020;2(2):53–61.
110. Somer E, Soffer-Dudek N, Ross CA. The comorbidity of daydreaming disorder (maladaptive daydreaming). J Nerv Ment Dis. 2017;205(7):525–30.
111. Soffer-Dudek N, Somer E, Spiegel D, Chefetz R, O'Neil J, Dorahy MJ, et al. Maladaptive daydreaming should be included as a dissociative disorder in psychiatric manuals: position paper. Br J Psychiatry. 2025;2025:1–5.
112. Bohus M, Stoffers-Winterling J, Sharp C, Krause-Utz A, Schmahl C, Lieb K. Borderline personality disorder. Lancet. 2021;398(10310):1528–40.
113. Crowell SE, Beauchaine TP, Linehan MM. A biosocial developmental model of borderline personality: elaborating and extending Linehan's theory. Psychol Bull. 2009;135(3):495–510.
114. Eaton NR, Greene AL. Personality disorders: community prevalence and socio-demographic correlates. Curr Opin Psychol. 2018;21:28–32.
115. Ellison WD, Rosenstein LK, Morgan TA, Zimmerman M. Community and clinical epidemiology of borderline personality disorder. Psychiatr Clin North Am. 2018;41(4):561–73.
116. Frías Á, Palma C. Comorbidity between post-traumatic stress disorder and borderline personality disorder: a review. Psychopathology. 2015;48(1):1–10.
117. Tomko RL, Trull TJ, Wood PK, Sher KJ. Characteristics of borderline personality disorder in a community sample: comorbidity, treatment utilization, and general functioning. J Pers Disord. 2014;28(5):734–50.
118. Pagura J, Stein MB, Bolton JM, Cox BJ, Grant B, Sareen J. Comorbidity of borderline personality disorder and posttraumatic stress disorder in the US population. J Psychiatric Res. 2010;44(16):1190–8.
119. Fornaro M, Orsolini L, Marini S, De Berardis D, Perna G, Valchera A, et al. The prevalence and predictors of bipolar and borderline personality disorders comorbidity: Systematic review and meta-analysis. J Affect Disord. 2016;195:105–18.

120. Philipsen A, Feige B, Hesslinger B, Scheel C, Ebert D, Matthies S, et al. Borderline typical symptoms in adult patients with attention deficit/hyperactivity disorder. Atten Defic Hyperact Disord. 2009;1(1):11–8.
121. Wertz J, Caspi A, Ambler A, Arseneault L, Belsky DW, Danese A, et al. Borderline symptoms at age 12 signal risk for poor outcomes during the transition to adulthood: findings from a genetically sensitive longitudinal cohort study. J Am Acad Child Adolesc Psychiatry. 2020;59(10):1165-1177.e2.
122. Chanen A, Sharp C, Hoffman P. Prevention and early intervention for borderline personality disorder: a novel public health priority. World Psychiatry. 2017;16(2):215–6.
123. Winsper C, Marwaha S, Lereya ST, Thompson A, Eyden J, Singh SP. Clinical and psychosocial outcomes of borderline personality disorder in childhood and adolescence: a systematic review. Psychol Med. 2015;45(11):2237–51.
124. Álvarez-Tomás I, Ruiz J, Guilera G, Bados A. Long-term clinical and functional course of borderline personality disorder: a meta-analysis of prospective studies. Eur Psychiatry. 2019;56:75–83.
125. Zanarini MC, Frankenburg FR, Reich DB, Wedig MM, Conkey LC, Fitzmaurice GM. The course of marriage/sustained cohabitation and parenthood among borderline patients followed prospectively for 16 years. J Pers Disord. 2015;29(1):62–70.
126. Temes CM, Zanarini MC. The longitudinal course of borderline personality disorder. Psychiatr Clin North Am. 2018;41(4):685–94.
127. Storebo OJ, Stoffers-Winterling JM, Vollm BA, Kongerslev MT, Mattivi JT, Jorgensen MS, et al. Psychological therapies for people with borderline personality disorder. Cochrane Database Syst Rev. 2020;2020(5):CD012955.
128. Zahediabghari S, Boursiquot P, Links P. Impact of psychotherapy on psychosocial functioning in borderline personality disorder patients. IJERPH. 2020;17(12):4610.
129. Bailey RC, Grenyer BFS. Supporting a person with personality disorder: a study of carer burden and well-being. J Pers Disord. 2014;28(6):796–809.
130. Grenyer BFS, Bailey RC, Lewis KL, Matthias M, Garretty T, Bickerton A. A randomized controlled trial of group psychoeducation for carers of persons with borderline personality disorder. J Pers Disord. 2019;33(2):214–28.
131. Guillen V, Diaz-Garcia A, Mira A, Garcia-Palacios A, Escriva-Martinez T, Banos R, et al. Interventions for family members and carers of patients with borderline personality disorder: a systematic review. Fam Process. 2020;2020:1.
132. Widiger TA, McCabe GA. The alternative model of personality disorders (AMPD) from the perspective of the five-factor model. Psychopathology. 2020;53(3–4):149–56.
133. Krueger RF, Hobbs KA. An overview of the DSM-5 alternative model of personality disorders. Psychopathology. 2020;53(3–4):126–32.

134. Alfieri M, Leucci AC, Bortolotti B, Gibiino S, Lia L, Pelizza L, et al. Dissociation and dysfunctional personality traits in patients with borderline personality disorder: a study based on DSM-5 alternative model. Eur J Psychiatry. 2025;39(1): 100283.
135. Tedesco V, Day NJS, Lucas S, Grenyer BFS. Diagnosing borderline personality disorder: reports and recommendations from people with lived experience. Personal Ment Health. 2024;18(2):107–21.
136. Zanarini MC, Frankenburg FR, Jager-Hyman S, Reich DB, Fitzmaurice G. The course of dissociation for patients with borderline personality disorder and axis II comparison subjects: a 10-year follow-up study. Acta Psychiatr Scand. 2008;118(4):291–6.
137. Niesten IJM, Glass IV, Zanarini MC. Course and prediction of dissociation in patients with borderline personality disorder and personality-disordered comparison subjects: a 24-year follow-up study. J Trauma Dissociation. 2024;2024:1–15.
138. Shah R, Zanarini MC. Comorbidity of borderline personality disorder: current status and future directions. Psychiatr Clin North Am. 2018;41(4):583–93.
139. Ross CA, Ferrell L, Schroeder E. Co-occurrence of dissociative identity disorder and borderline personality disorder. J Trauma Dissociation. 2014;15(1):79–90.
140. Antoine SM, Fredborg BK, Streiner D, Guimond T, Dixon-Gordon KL, Chapman AL, et al. Subgroups of borderline personality disorder: a latent class analysis. Psychiatry Res. 2023;323: 115131.
141. Kaess M. Childhood adversity in borderline personality disorder—a call for a more systemic approach to early intervention and prevention. Acta Psychiatr Scand. 2020;141(1):3–5.
142. Goldbach RE, Neukel C, Panizza A, Reinken A, Krause-Utz A. Differentiating between intrapsychic symptoms and behavioral expressions of borderline personality disorder in relation to childhood emotional maltreatment and emotion dysregulation: an exploratory investigation. Eur J Psychotraumatol. 2023;14(2):2263317.
143. Lynch TR, Hempel RJ, Dunkley C. Radically open-dialectical behavior therapy for disorders of over-control: signaling matters. Am J Psychother. 2015;69(2):141–62.
144. Miller CE, Townsend ML, Grenyer BFS. Understanding chronic feelings of emptiness in borderline personality disorder: a qualitative study. Borderline Personal Disord Emot Dysregul. 2021;8(1):24.
145. Powers A, Petri JM, Sleep C, Mekawi Y, Lathan EC, Shebuski K, et al. Distinguishing PTSD, complex PTSD, and borderline personality disorder using exploratory structural equation modeling in a trauma-exposed urban sample. J Anxiety Disord. 2022;88: 102558.

146. Porter C, Palmier-Claus J, Branitsky A, Mansell W, Warwick H, Varese F. Childhood adversity and borderline personality disorder: a meta-analysis. Acta Psychiatr Scand. 2020;141(1):6–20.
147. Jowett S, Karatzias T, Shevlin M, Albert I. Differentiating symptom profiles of ICD-11 PTSD, complex PTSD, and borderline personality disorder: a latent class analysis in a multiply traumatized sample. Personal Disord Theory Res Treat. 2020;11(1):36–45.
148. Hyland P, Karatzias T, Shevlin M, Cloitre M. Examining the discriminant validity of complex posttraumatic stress disorder and borderline personality disorder symptoms: results from a United Kingdom population sample. J Trauma Stress. 2019;32(6):855–63.
149. Frost R, Hyland P, Shevlin M, Murphy J. Distinguishing complex PTSD from borderline personality disorder among individuals with a history of sexual trauma: a latent class analysis. Eur J Trauma Dissociation. 2020;4(1): 100080.
150. Tschoeke S, Steinert T, Knoblauch H. Forensic aspects of dissociative positive symptoms in trauma-related disorders and borderline personality disorder. Int J Law Psychiatry. 2024;94: 101973.
151. Arroyo Sánchez E, Setién PP. Differential diagnosis of psychosis and dissociative disorder: a case report. Eur Psychiatr. 2023;66(S1):S750–S750.
152. Beatson JA, Broadbear JH, Duncan C, Bourton D, Rao S. Avoiding misdiagnosis when auditory verbal hallucinations are present in borderline personality disorder. J Nerv Ment Dis. 2019;207(12):1048–55.
153. Slotema CW, Blom JD, Niemantsverdriet MBA, Sommer IEC. Auditory verbal hallucinations in borderline personality disorder and the efficacy of antipsychotics: a systematic review. Front Psychiatry. 2018;31(9):347.
154. Longden E, Branitsky A, Moskowitz A, Berry K, Bucci S, Varese F. The relationship between dissociation and symptoms of psychosis: a meta-analysis. Schizophr Bull. 2020;46(5):1104–13.
155. Pietkiewicz IJ, Tomalski R, Hełka AM. Developing a codebook for assessing auditory hallucination complexity using mixed methods. Front Psychiatry. 2024;15:1441919.
156. Schäfer I, Langeland W, Hissbach J, Luedecke C, Ohlmeier MD, Chodzinski C, et al. Childhood trauma and dissociation in patients with alcohol dependence, drug dependence, or both—a multi-center study. Drug Alcohol Depend. 2010;109(1–3):84–9.
157. Najavits LM, Walsh M. Dissociation, PTSD, and substance abuse: an empirical study. J Trauma Dissociation. 2012;13(1):115–26.
158. Klanecky A, McChargue DE, Bruggeman L. Desire to dissociate: implications for problematic drinking in college students with childhood or adolescent sexual abuse exposure. Am J Addict. 2012;21(3):250–6.

159. Craparo G, Ardino V, Gori A, Caretti V. The relationships between early trauma, dissociation, and alexithymia in alcohol addiction. Psychiatry Investig. 2014;11(3):330.
160. Schäfer I, Reininghaus U, Langeland W, Voss A, Zieger N, Haasen C, et al. Dissociative symptoms in alcohol-dependent patients: associations with childhood trauma and substance abuse characteristics. Compr Psychiatry. 2007;48(6):539–45.
161. Ricci V, Ceci F, Di Carlo F, Lalli A, Ciavoni L, Mosca A, et al. Cannabis use disorder and dissociation: a report from a prospective first-episode psychosis study. Drug Alcohol Depend. 2021;229: 109118.
162. Good MI. Substance-induced dissociative disorders and psychiatric nosology. J Clin Psychopharmacol. 1989;9(2):88–93.
163. Somer E, Altus L, Ginzburg K. Dissociative psychopathology among opioid use disorder patients: exploring the "chemical dissociation" hypothesis. Compr Psychiatry. 2010;51(4):419–25.
164. Van Heugten-Van Der Kloet D, Giesbrecht T, Van Wel J, Bosker WM, Kuypers KP, Theunissen EL, et al. MDMA, cannabis, and cocaine produce acute dissociative symptoms. Psychiatry Res. 2015;228(3):907–12.
165. Castle C, Gray A, Neehoff S, Glue P. Effect of ketamine dose on self-rated dissociation in patients with treatment refractory anxiety disorders. J Psychopharmacol. 2017;31(10):1306–11.
166. Danböck SK, Duek O, Ben-Zion Z, Korem N, Amen SL, Kelmendi B, et al. Effects of a dissociative drug on fronto-limbic resting-state functional connectivity in individuals with posttraumatic stress disorder: a randomized controlled pilot study. Psychopharmacology. 2024;241(2):243–52.
167. Thal SB, Daniels JK, Jungaberle H. The link between childhood trauma and dissociation in frequent users of classic psychedelics and dissociatives. J Substance Use. 2019;24(5):524–31.
168. Brand BL, Lanius R, Vermetten E, Loewenstein RJ, Spiegel D. Where are we going? an update on assessment, treatment, and neurobiological research in dissociative disorders as we move toward the *DSM-5*. J Trauma Dissociation. 2012;13(1):9–31.
169. International Society For The Study. Guidelines for treating dissociative identity disorder in adults, third revision. J Trauma Dissociation. 2011;12(2):115–87.
170. Coy DM, Madere JA. Diagnosing the dissociative disorders: Conceptual, theoretical, and practical considerations. In: Dorahy MJ, Gold SN, O'Neil JA, editors. Dissociation and the dissociative disorders: past, present, future. 2nd ed. Routledge; 2023. p. 661–72.
171. Wainipitapong S, Millman LSM, Huang X, Wieder L, Terhune DB, Pick S. Assessing dissociation: a systematic review and evaluation of existing measures. J Psychiatr Res. 2024;181:91–8.

172. Steinberg M, Hall P. The SCID-D diagnostic interview and treatment planning in dissociative disorders. Bull Menninger Clin. 1997;61(1):108–20.
173. Ross CA, Heber S, Norton GR, Anderson D, Barcher P. The dissociative disorders interview schedule: a structured interview. Dissociation. Prog Dissociative Disord. 1989;2(3):169–89.
174. Bernstein EM, Putnam FW. Development, reliability, and validity of a dissociation scale. J Nerv Ment Dis. 1986;174(12):727–35.
175. Carlson EB, Putnam FW. An update on the dissociative experiences scale. Dissociation Prog Dissociative Disord. 1993;6(1):16–27.
176. Vanijzendoorn M, Schuengel C. The measurement of dissociation in normal and clinical populations: meta-analytic validation of the Dissociative Experiences Scale (DES). Clin Psychol Rev. 1996;16(5):365–82.
177. Sierra M, Berrios GE. The Cambridge depersonalization scale: a new instrument for the measurement of depersonalization. Psychiatry Res. 2000;93(2):153–64.
178. Vanderlinden J, Van Dyck R, Vandereycken W, Vertommen H, Jan VR. The dissociation questionnaire (DIS-Q): development and characteristics of a new self-report questionnaire. Clin Psychology and Psychoth. 1993;1(1):21–7.
179. Nijenhuis ERS, Spinhoven P, Van Dyck R, Der Hart OV, Vanderlinden J. The development and psychometric characteristics of the somatoform dissociation questionnaire (SDQ-20). J Nervous Ment Dis. 1996;184(11):688–94.
180. Bremner JD, Krystal JH, Putnam FW, Southwick SM, Marmar C, Charney DS, et al. Measurement of dissociative states with the clinician-administered dissociative states scale (CADSS). J Trauma Stress. 1998;11(1):125–36.
181. Mertens YL, Daniels JK. The clinician-administered dissociative states scale (CADSS): validation of the German version. J Trauma Dissociation. 2022;23(4):366–84.
182. Stiglmayr CE, Shapiro DA, Stieglitz RD, Limberger MF, Bohus M. Experience of aversive tension and dissociation in female patients with borderline personality disorder—a controlled study. J Psychiatr Res. 2001;35(2):111–8.
183. Stiglmayr C, Schmahl C, Bremner JD, Bohus M, Ebner-Priemer U. Development and psychometric characteristics of the DSS-4 as a short instrument to assess dissociative experience during neuropsychological experiments. Psychopathology. 2009;42(6):370–4.
184. Macia KS, Carlson EB, Palmieri PA, Smith SR, Anglin DM, Ghosh Ippen C, et al. Development of a brief version of the dissociative symptoms scale and the reliability and validity of DSS-B scores in diverse clinical and community samples. Assessment. 2023;30(7):2058–73.
185. Heekerens JB, Preece DA, Gross JJ. The Stanford dissociation questionnaire: a three-facet measure of trait and state dissociation.
186. Mychailyszyn MP, Brand BL, Webermann AR, Şar V, Draijer N. Differentiating dissociative from non-dissociative disorders: a meta-analysis of the

structured clinical interview for DSM dissociative disorders (SCID-D). J Trauma Dissociation. 2021;22(1):19–34.
187. Ross CA, Browning E. The self-report dissociative disorders interview schedule: a preliminary report. J Trauma Dissociation. 2017;18(1):31–7.
188. Eidhof MB, Ter Heide FJJ, Van Der Aa N, Schreckenbach M, Schmidt U, Brand BL, et al. The dissociative subtype of PTSD interview (DSP-I): development and psychometric properties. J Trauma Dissociation. 2019;20(5):564–81.
189. Weathers FW, Bovin MJ, Lee DJ, Sloan DM, Schnurr PP, Kaloupek DG, et al. The clinician-administered PTSD scale for DSM–5 (CAPS-5): development and initial psychometric evaluation in military veterans. Psychol Assess. 2018;30(3):383–95.
190. Niesten. Symptom over-reporting ≠ malingering: from faulty archetypes to a nuanced empirical perspective [Internet]. maastricht university; 2019 [cited 2025 June 23]. Available from: https://cris.maastrichtuniversity.nl/portal/en/publications/symptom-overreporting--malingering(6cc37a62-a50a-4ddc-91b0-185773db9842).html
191. Lynn SJ, Lilienfeld SO, Merckelbach H, Giesbrecht T, Van Der Kloet D. Dissociation and dissociative disorders: challenging conventional wisdom. Curr Dir Psychol Sci. 2012;21(1):48–53.
192. Cheung CTY, Cheng CMH, Lee VWP, Lam SKK, He KL, Ling HWH, et al. Could family well-being moderate the relationship between adverse childhood experiences and somatoform dissociation? A preliminary investigation. J Trauma Dissociation. 2024;25(2):153–67.
193. Sar V, Dorahy M, Krüger C. Revisiting the etiological aspects of dissociative identity disorder: a biopsychosocial perspective. PRBM. 2017;10:137–46.
194. Dissociation debates: everything you know is wrong. Dialogues Clin Neurosci. 2018;20(3):229–42.
195. Akwa-GGZ, Dutch Mental Health Care Standards: Dissociative disorders. 2020: Utrech [Internet]. Available from: https://www.ggzstandaarden.nl/zorgstandaarden/dissociatieve-stoornissen/introductie
196. Lynn SJ, Maxwell R, Merckelbach H, Lilienfeld SO, van Kloet DVHD, Miskovic V. Dissociation and its disorders: competing models, future directions, and a way forward. Clin Psychol Rev. 2019;73:101755.
197. Vonderlin R, Kleindienst N, Alpers GW, Bohus M, Lyssenko L, Schmahl C. Dissociation in victims of childhood abuse or neglect: a meta-analytic review. Psychol Med. 2018;48(15):2467–76.
198. Zanarini MC, Ruser TF, Frankenburg FR, Hennen J, Gunderson JG. Risk factors associated with the dissociative experiences of borderline patients. J Nerv Ment Dis. 2000;188(1):26–30.

199. Dalenberg CJ, Brand BL, Gleaves DH, Dorahy MJ, Loewenstein RJ, Cardeña E, et al. Evaluation of the evidence for the trauma and fantasy models of dissociation. Psychol Bull. 2012;138(3):550–88.
200. Dalenberg C, Naish B, Abu-Rus A. Dissociation, Dissociative Disorder, and Their Treatment. In: Geffner R, White JW, Hamberger LK, Rosenbaum A, Vaughan-Eden V, Vieth VI, editors. Handbook of Interpersonal Violence and Abuse Across the Lifespan [Internet]. Cham: Springer International Publishing; 2022 [cited 2024 July 15]. p. 4383–408. Available from: https://link.springer.com/https://doi.org/10.1007/978-3-319-89999-2_177
201. Boyer SM, Caplan JE, Edwards LK. Trauma-related dissociation and the dissociative disorders: delaware. J Public Health. 2022;8(2):78–84.
202. Rafiq S, Campodonico C, Varese F. The relationship between childhood adversities and dissociation in severe mental illness: a meta-analytic review. Acta Psychiatr Scand. 2018;138(6):509–25.
203. Vonderlin R, Kleindienst N, Alpers GW, Bohus M, Lyssenko L, Schmahl C. Dissociation in victims of childhood abuse or neglect: a meta-analytic review. Psychol Med. 2018;48(15):2467–76.
204. Frewen PA, Lanius RA. Trauma-related altered states of consciousness: exploring the 4-D model. J Trauma Dissociation. 2014;15(4):436–56.
205. Lanius RA, Vermetten E, Loewenstein RJ, Brand B, Schmahl C, Bremner JD, et al. Emotion modulation in PTSD: clinical and neurobiological evidence for a dissociative subtype. AJP. 2010;167(6):640–7.
206. Lanius RA. Trauma-related dissociation and altered states of consciousness: a call for clinical, treatment, and neuroscience research. Eur J Psychotraumatol. 2015;6(1):27905.
207. Briere J, Hodges M, Godbout N. Traumatic stress, affect dysregulation, and dysfunctional avoidance: a structural equation model. J Trauma Stress. 2010;23(6):767–74.
208. Brewin CR, Dalgleish T, Joseph S. A dual representation theory of posttraumatic stress disorder. Psychol Rev. 1996;103(4):670–86.
209. Berntsen D, Nielsen NP. The reconstructive nature of involuntary autobiographical memories. Memory. 2022;30(1):31–6.
210. Bedard-Gilligan M, Zoellner LA. Dissociation and memory fragmentation in post-traumatic stress disorder: an evaluation of the dissociative encoding hypothesis. Memory. 2012;20(3):277–99.
211. Thompson-Hollands J, Jun JJ, Sloan DM. The association between peritraumatic dissociation and PTSD symptoms: the mediating role of negative beliefs about the self. J Trauma Stress. 2017;30(2):190–4.
212. Burback L, Forner C, Winkler O, Al-Shamali H, Ayoub Y, Paquet J, et al. Survival, attachment, and healing: an evolutionary lens on interventions for trauma-related dissociation. PRBM. 2024;17:2403–31.

213. Schauer M, Elbert T. Dissociation following traumatic stress: etiology and treatment. Z Psychol J Psychol. 2010;218(2):109–27.
214. Beutler S, Mertens YL, Ladner L, Schellong J, Croy I, Daniels JK. Trauma-related dissociation and the autonomic nervous system: a systematic literature review of psychophysiological correlates of dissociative experiencing in PTSD patients. Eur J Psychotraumatol. 2022;13(2):2132599.
215. Kumpula MJ, Orcutt HK, Bardeen JR, Varkovitzky RL. Peritraumatic dissociation and experiential avoidance as prospective predictors of posttraumatic stress symptoms. J Abnorm Psychol. 2011;120(3):617–27.
216. Putnam FW. Dissociative disorders in children: behavioral profiles and problems. Child Abuse Negl. 1993;17(1):39–45.
217. Lyons-Ruth K, Dutra L, Schuder MR, Bianchi I. From infant attachment disorganization to adult dissociation: Relational adaptations or traumatic experiences? Psychiatr Clin North Am. 2006;29(1):63–86.
218. Heim C, Nemeroff CB. The role of childhood trauma in the neurobiology of mood and anxiety disorders: preclinical and clinical studies. Biol Psychiat. 2001;49(12):1023–39.
219. Teicher MH, Samson JA. Annual research review: enduring neurobiological effects of childhood abuse and neglect. J Child Psychol Psychiatr. 2016;57(3):241–66.
220. Cicchetti D. Gene-environment interaction. Dev Psychopathol. 2007;19(4):957–9.
221. Sroufe LA. The concept of development in developmental psychopathology. Child Dev Perspect. 2009;3(3):178–83.
222. Luyten P, Campbell C, Fonagy P. Rethinking the relationship between attachment and personality disorder. Curr Opin Psychol. 2021;37:109–13.
223. Kernberg OF. Severe personality disorders. New Haven: Yale University Press; 1984.
224. Guérin-Marion C, Sezlik S, Bureau JF. Developmental and attachment-based perspectives on dissociation: beyond the effects of maltreatment. Eur J Psychotraumatol. 2020;11(1):1802908.
225. Carlson EB, Palmieri PA, Field NP, Dalenberg CJ, Macia KS, Spain DA. Contributions of risk and protective factors to prediction of psychological symptoms after traumatic experiences. Compr Psychiatry. 2016;69:106–15.
226. Kyron MJ, Rees CS, Lawrence D, Carleton RN, McEvoy PM. Prospective risk and protective factors for psychopathology and wellbeing in civilian emergency services personnel: a systematic review. J Affect Disord. 2021;281:517–32.
227. Bowlby J. Attachment and loss, vol. 1. New York: Basic Books; 1969.
228. Ainsworth MD, Bell SM. Attachment, exploration, and separation: illustrated by the behavior of one-year-olds in a strange situation. Child Dev. 1970;41(1):49–67.

229. Karatzias T, Shevlin M, Ford JD, Fyvie C, Grandison G, Hyland P, et al. Childhood trauma, attachment orientation, and complex PTSD (CPTSD) symptoms in a clinical sample: Implications for treatment. Dev Psychopathol. 2022;34(3):1192–7.
230. Godbout N, Daspe MÈ, Runtz M, Cyr G, Briere J. Childhood maltreatment, attachment, and borderline personality–related symptoms: gender-specific structural equation models. Psychol Trauma Theory Res Pract Policy. 2019;11(1):90–8.
231. Zajac K, Kobak R. Caregiver unresolved loss and abuse and child behavior problems: intergenerational effects in a high-risk sample. Dev Psychopathol. 2009;21(1):173–87.
232. Greene CA, Haisley L, Wallace C, Ford JD. Intergenerational effects of childhood maltreatment: a systematic review of the parenting practices of adult survivors of childhood abuse, neglect, and violence. Clin Psychol Rev. 2020;80: 101891.
233. Rimmington D, Roberts R, Sawyer A, Sved-Williams A. Dissociation in mothers with borderline personality disorder: a possible mechanism for transmission of intergenerational trauma? A scoping review. Bord Personal Disord Emot Dysregul. 2024;11(1):7.
234. Byun S, Brumariu LE, Lyons-Ruth K. Disorganized attachment in young adulthood as a partial mediator of relations between severity of childhood abuse and dissociation. J Trauma Dissociation. 2016;17(4):460–79.
235. Hébert M, Langevin R, Charest F. Disorganized attachment and emotion dysregulation as mediators of the association between sexual abuse and dissociation in preschoolers. J Affect Disord. 2020;267:220–8.
236. Rüfenacht E, Shaverin L, Stubley J, Smits ML, Bateman A, Fonagy P, et al. Addressing dissociation symptoms with trauma-focused mentalization-based treatment. Psychoanal Psychother. 2023;37(4):467–91.
237. Bateman A, Rüfenacht E, Perroud N, Debbané M, Nolte T, Shaverin L, et al. Childhood maltreatment, dissociation and borderline personality disorder: Preliminary data on the mediational role of mentalizing in complex post-traumatic stress disorder. Psychol Psychother. 2023;2023, papt.12514.
238. Luyten P, Campbell C, Allison E, Fonagy P. The Mentalizing Approach to Psychopathology: State of the Art and Future Directions. Annu Rev Clin Psychol. 2020;16:297–325.
239. Gobin RL, Freyd JJ. The impact of betrayal trauma on the tendency to trust. Psychol Trauma Theory Res Pract Policy. 2014;6(5):505–11.
240. Bateman A, Fonagy P. Mentalization based treatment for borderline personality disorder. World Psychiatry. 2010;9(1):11–5.
241. Nijenhuis E, Van Der Hart O, Steele K. Trauma-related structural dissociation of the personality. Act Nerv Super. 2010;52(1):1–23.

242. Zhu J, Exner-Cortens D, Dobson K, Wells L, Noel M, Madigan S. Adverse childhood experiences and intimate partner violence: a meta-analysis. Dev Psychopathol. 2024;36(2):929–43.
243. Li S, Zhao F, Yu G. Childhood maltreatment and intimate partner violence victimization: a meta-analysis. Child Abuse Negl. 2019;88:212–24.
244. Capaldi DM, Knoble NB, Shortt JW, Kim HK. A systematic review of risk factors for intimate partner violence. Partn Abus. 2012;3(2):231–80.
245. Fereidooni F, Daniels JK, D Krause-Utz A, Hagenaars MA, Smeets T, Heins J, et al. Childhood maltreatment and adulthood victimization: an evidence-based model. J Psychiatr Res. 2023;167:46–62.
246. Noll JG, Horowitz LA, Bonanno GA, Trickett PK, Putnam FW. Revictimization and self-harm in females who experienced childhood sexual abuse: results from a prospective study. J Interpers Violence. 2003;18(12):1452–71.
247. Scoglio AAJ, Kraus SW, Saczynski J, Jooma S, Molnar BE. Systematic review of risk and protective factors for revictimization after child sexual abuse. Trauma Violence Abuse. 2021;22(1):41–53.
248. Widom CS, Czaja SJ, Dutton MA. Childhood victimization and lifetime revictimization. Child Abuse Negl. 2008;32(8):785–96.
249. Zamir O, Szepsenwol O, Englund MM, Simpson JA. The role of dissociation in revictimization across the lifespan: a 32-year prospective study. Child Abuse Negl. 2018;79:144–53.
250. Noll JG, Horowitz LA, Bonanno GA, Trickett PK, Putnam FW. Revictimization and self-harm in females who experienced childhood sexual abuse: results from a prospective study. J Interpers Violence. 2003;18(12):1452–71.
251. de Waal MM, Christ C, Messman TL, Dekker JJM. Changes in Risk Perception After Sexual Victimization: Are We Following the Right Track? J Interpers Violence. 2022;37(13–14):NP11699–719.
252. Bockers E, Roepke S, Michael L, Renneberg B, Knaevelsrud C. Risk recognition, attachment anxiety, self-efficacy, and state dissociation predict revictimization. PLoS ONE. 2014;9(9): e108206.
253. Kulacaoglu F, Solmaz M, Ardic FC, Akin E, Kose S. The relationship between childhood traumas, dissociation, and impulsivity in patients with borderline personality disorder comorbid with ADHD. Psychiatry Clin Psychopharmacol. 2017;27(4):393–402.
254. Somer E, Ginzburg K, Kramer L. The role of impulsivity in the association between childhood trauma and dissociative psychopathology: mediation versus moderation. Psychiatry Res. 2012;196(1):133–7.
255. Webermann AR, Brand BL. Mental illness and violent behavior: the role of dissociation. Bord Personal Disord Emot Dysregul. 2017;4(1):2.

256. Webermann AR, Myrick AC, Taylor CL, Chasson GS, Brand BL. Dissociative, depressive, and PTSD symptom severity as correlates of nonsuicidal self-injury and suicidality in dissociative disorder patients. J Trauma Dissociation. 2016;17(1):67–80.
257. Basso JC, Satyal MK, McKee KL, Lynn S, Gyamfi D, Bickel WK. Dissociation and other trauma symptomatology are linked to imbalance in the competing neurobehavioral decision systems. Front Psychol. 2024;14:1317088.
258. Harris A, Gous G, de Wet B, Griffiths MD. The relationship between gambling event frequency, motor response inhibition, arousal, and dissociative experience. J Gambl Stud. 2021;37(1):241–68.
259. Krause-Utz A, Steinmann S, German M, Piccioni-Grenna S, Ende G, Schmahl C. Impact of acute dissociation on behavioural impulsivity under stress conditions in borderline personality disorder and attention deficit hyperactivity disorder: associations with childhood trauma. In preparation.
260. Krause-Utz A, Dierick T, Josef T, Chatzaki E, Willem A, Hoogenboom J, et al. Linking experiences of child sexual abuse to adult sexual intimate partner violence: the role of borderline personality features, maladaptive cognitive emotion regulation, and dissociation. Borderline Personal Disord Emot Dysregul. 2021;8(1):10.
261. Sugg N. Intimate partner violence. Med Clin North Am. 2015;99(3):629–49.
262. Whitaker DJ, Haileyesus T, Swahn M, Saltzman LS. Differences in frequency of violence and reported injury between relationships with reciprocal and nonreciprocal intimate partner violence. Am J Public Health. 2007;97(5):941–7.
263. Webermann AR, Murphy CM. Childhood trauma and dissociative intimate partner violence. Violence Against Women. 2019;25(2):148–66.
264. Krause-Utz A, Černáková R, Hoogenboom W, Schulze A, Büttner S, Demirelli Z, et al. Psychological factors linked to intimate partner violence and childhood maltreatment: on dissociation as a possible bridge symptom. J Interpers Violence. 2023;38(21–22):11400–28.
265. Pilkington P, Younan R, Bishop A. Early maladaptive schemas, suicidal ideation, and self-harm: a meta-analytic review. J Affect Disorders Rep. 2021;3: 100051.
266. Dutton DG, White KR. Attachment insecurity and intimate partner violence. Aggress Violent Beh. 2012;17(5):475–81.
267. Whitaker DJ, Haileyesus T, Swahn M, Saltzman LS. Differences in frequency of violence and reported injury between relationships with reciprocal and nonreciprocal intimate partner violence. Am J Public Health. 2007;97(5):941–7.

268. Sabri B, Simonet M, Campbell JC. Risk and protective factors of intimate partner violence among South Asian immigrant women and perceived need for services. Cultur Divers Ethnic Minor Psychol. 2018;24(3):442–52.
269. Ortega Pacheco YJ, Gallo-Barrera YD, Pozo MC. Risk and protective factors for revictimization from intimate partner violence: a systematic review. Int J Soc Psychiatry. 2024;70(8):1379–91.
270. Hoeboer CM, De Kleine RA, Molendijk ML, Schoorl M, Oprel DAC, Mouthaan J, et al. Impact of dissociation on the effectiveness of psychotherapy for post-traumatic stress disorder: meta-analysis. BJPsych Open. 2020;6(3):e53.
271. Ebner-Priemer UW, Mauchnik J, Kleindienst N, Schmahl C, Peper M, Rosenthal MZ, et al. Emotional learning during dissociative states in borderline personality disorder. J Psychiatry Neurosci. 2009;34(3):214–22.
272. Post-traumatic stress disorder. NICE guideline [Internet]. 2018. Available from: www.nice.org.uk/guidance/ng116
273. Winter D, Krause-Utz A, Lis S, Chiu CD, Lanius RA, Schriner F, et al. Dissociation in borderline personality disorder: disturbed cognitive and emotional inhibition and its neural correlates. Psychiatry Res Neuroimaging. 2015;233(3):339–51.
274. Karatzias T, Murphy P, Cloitre M, Bisson J, Roberts N, Shevlin M, et al. Psychological interventions for ICD-11 complex PTSD symptoms: systematic review and meta-analysis. Psychol Med. 2019;49(11):1761–75.
275. Lanius RA, Brand B, Vermetten E, Frewen PA, Spiegel D. The dissociative subtype of posttraumatic stress disorder: rationale, clinical and neurobiological evidence, and implications: dissociative subtype of PTSD. Depress Anxiety. 2012;29(8):701–8.
276. Haagen JFG, Van Rijn A, Knipscheer JW, Van Der Aa N, Kleber RJ. The dissociative post-traumatic stress disorder (PTSD) subtype: a treatment outcome cohort study in veterans with PTSD. Br J Clinic Psychol. 2018;57(2):203–22.
277. van Heugten-van der Kloet D, Huntjens R, Giesbrecht T, Merckelbach H. Self-reported sleep disturbances in patients with dissociative identity disorder and post-traumatic stress disorder and how they relate to cognitive failures and fantasy proneness. Front Psychiatry [Internet]. 2014 [cited 2020 Nov 21];5. Available from: https://doi.org/10.3389/fpsyt.2014.00019/abstract.
278. Lilienfeld SO, Kirsch I, Sarbin TR, Lynn SJ, Chaves JF, Ganaway GK, et al. Dissociative identity disorder and the sociocognitive model: recalling the lessons of the past. Psychol Bull. 1999;125(5):507–23.
279. Zerubavel N, Messman-Moore TL. Staying present: incorporating mindfulness into therapy for dissociation. Mindfulness. 2015;6(2):303–14.
280. Bregman-Hai N, Abitbul-Gordon S, Deutsch I, Garbi D, Shelef L, Soffer-Dudek N. Leave everything to the imagination: cognitive functioning of

individuals high in dissociative absorption and imaginative involvement. J Res Pers. 2018;76:129–38.
281. Giesbrecht T, Lynn SJ, Lilienfeld SO, Merckelbach H. Cognitive processes in dissociation: an analysis of core theoretical assumptions. Psychol Bull. 2008;134(5):617–47.
282. Huntjens RJC, Janssen GPJ, Merckelbach H, Lynn SJ. The link between dissociative tendencies and hyperassociativity. J Behav Ther Exp Psychiatry. 2021;73: 101665.
283. Vissia EM, Lawrence AJ, Chalavi S, Giesen ME, Draijer N, Nijenhuis ERS, et al. Dissociative identity state-dependent working memory in dissociative identity disorder: a controlled functional magnetic resonance imaging study. BJPsych open. 2022;8(3): e82.
284. Spanos NP. Multiple identity enactments and multiple personality disorder: a sociocognitive perspective. Psychol Bull. 1994;116(1):143–65.
285. Dell PF. Reconsidering the autohypnotic model of the dissociative disorders. J Trauma Dissociation. 2019;20(1):48–78.
286. Koffel E, Watson D. Unusual sleep experiences, dissociation, and schizotypy: evidence for a common domain. Clin Psychol Rev. 2009;29(6):548–59.
287. Watson D. Dissociations of the night: Individual differences in sleep-related experiences and their relation to dissociation and schizotypy. J Abnorm Psychol. 2001;110(4):526–35.
288. Soffer-Dudek N. Arousal in nocturnal consciousness: how dream- and sleep-experiences may inform us of poor sleep quality, stress, and psychopathology. Front Psychol. 2017;8:733.
289. Arora T, Alhelali E, Grey I. Poor sleep efficiency and daytime napping are risk factors of depersonalization disorder in female university students. Neurobiol Sleep Circ Rhythms. 2020;9: 100059.
290. van Heugten-van der Kloet D, Giesbrecht T, Merckelbach H. Sleep loss increases dissociation and affects memory for emotional stimuli. J Behav Ther Exp Psychiatry. 2015;47:9–17.
291. Dimitrova L, Fernando V, Vissia EM, Nijenhuis ERS, Draijer N, Reinders AATS. Sleep, trauma, fantasy and cognition in dissociative identity disorder, post-traumatic stress disorder and healthy controls: a replication and extension study. Eur J Psychotraumatol. 2020;11(1):1705599.
292. Gratz KL, Roemer L. Multidimensional assessment of emotion regulation and dysregulation: development, factor structure, and initial validation of the difficulties in emotion regulation scale. J Psychopathol Behav Assess. 2004;26(1):41–54.
293. Girme YU, Jones RE, Fleck C, Simpson JA, Overall NC. Infants' attachment insecurity predicts attachment-relevant emotion regulation strategies in adulthood. Emotion. 2021;21(2):260–72.

294. New AS, Rot M aan het, Ripoll LH, Perez-Rodriguez MM, Lazarus S, Zipursky E, et al. Empathy and alexithymia in borderline personality disorder: clinical and laboratory measures. J Personality Disord. 2012;26(5):660–75.
295. Rudy JA, McKernan S, Kouri N, D'Andrea W. A meta-analysis of the association between shame and dissociation. J Trauma Stress. 2022;35(5):1318–33.
296. Cavicchioli M, Scalabrini A, Northoff G, Mucci C, Ogliari A, Maffei C. Dissociation and emotion regulation strategies: a meta-analytic review. J Psychiatr Res. 2021;143:370–87.
297. Cavicchioli M, Ogliari A, Maffei C, Mucci C, Scalabrini A. Dissociative dimensions and their implications for emotional dysregulation underlying borderline personality disorder features. J Nerv Ment Dis. 2023;211(10):742–51.
298. Reyno SM, Simmons M, Kinley J. A meta-analytic study examining the relationship between alexithymia and dissociation in psychiatric and non-clinical populations. ResPsy [Internet]. 2020 May 21 [cited 2025 Jan 22];23(1). Available from: https://www.researchinpsychotherapy.org/index.php/rpsy/article/view/439.
299. Van Der Kolk B, Ford JD, Spinazzola J. Comorbidity of developmental trauma disorder (DTD) and post-traumatic stress disorder: findings from the DTD field trial. Eur J Psychotraumatol. 2019;10(1):1562841.
300. Wise TN, Mann LS, Sheridan MJ. Relationship between alexithymia, dissociation and personality in psychiatric outpatients. Psychother Psychosom. 2000;69(3):123–7.
301. Young JE, Klosko JS, Weishaar ME. Schema therapy: a practitioner's guide. New York: Guilford Press; 2003.
302. Johnston C, Dorahy MJ, Courtney D, Bayles T, O'Kane M. Dysfunctional schema modes, childhood trauma and dissociation in borderline personality disorder. J Behav Ther Exp Psychiatry. 2009;40(2):248–55.
303. Van Der Linde RPA, Huntjens RJC, Bachrach N, Rijkeboer MM. Personality disorder traits, maladaptive schemas, modes and coping styles in participants with complex dissociative disorders, borderline personality disorder and avoidant personality disorder. Clin Psychology Psychoth. 2023;30(6):1234–45.
304. Tan YM, Lee CW, Averbeck LE, Brand-de Wilde O, Farrell J, Fassbinder E, et al. Schema therapy for borderline personality disorder: a qualitative study of patients' perceptions. PLoS ONE. 2018;13(11): e0206039.
305. Blackman LC, Pizarro-Campagna E, Pilkington PD. Early maladaptive schemas and dissociative symptoms: a systematic review and meta-analysis. Clin Psychol Psychother. 2024;31(6): e70026.

306. Khosravi M. Child maltreatment-related dissociation and its core mediation schemas in patients with borderline personality disorder. BMC Psychiatry. 2020;20(1):405.
307. Wright MO, Crawford E, Del Castillo D. Childhood emotional maltreatment and later psychological distress among college students: the mediating role of maladaptive schemas. Child Abuse Negl. 2009;33(1):59–68.
308. Schimmenti A. Dissociative experiences and dissociative minds: Exploring a nomological network of dissociative functioning. J Trauma Dissociation. 2016;17(3):338–61.
309. Sempértegui GA, Karreman A, Arntz A, Bekker MHJ. Schema therapy for borderline personality disorder: a comprehensive review of its empirical foundations, effectiveness and implementation possibilities. Clin Psychol Rev. 2013;33(3):426–47.
310. Barazandeh H, Kissane David W, Saeedi N, Gordon M. Schema modes and dissociation in borderline personality disorder/traits in adolescents or young adults. Psychiatry Res. 2018;261:1–6.
311. Borsboom D, Cramer AOJ. Network analysis: an integrative approach to the structure of psychopathology. Annu Rev Clin Psychol. 2013;9(1):91–121.
312. Heekerens JB, Schulze L, Enge J, Renneberg B, Roepke S. Affective arousal temporally precedes dissociation in patients with borderline personality disorder: a preliminary experience sampling study. Psychological Trauma: Theory, Research, Practice, and Policy [Internet]. 2023 May 1 [cited 2024 July 18]; Available from: https://doi.org/10.1037/tra0001516.
313. Stiglmayr CE, Ebner-Priemer UW, Bretz J, Behm R, Mohse M, Lammers C-H, et al. Dissociative symptoms are positively related to stress in borderline personality disorder. Acta Psychiatr Scand. 2008;117(2):139–47.
314. Fatimah H, Rappaport LM, Bornovalova MA. Symptoms of borderline personality and related pathologies behave as temporal and contemporaneous networks. Personal Disord Theory Res Treat. 2023;14(4):467–77.
315. Graumann L, Heekerens JB, Duesenberg M, Metz S, Spitzer C, Otte C, et al. Association between baseline dissociation levels and stress-induced state dissociation in patients with posttraumatic-stress disorder, borderline personality disorder, and major depressive disorder. Borderline Personal Disord Emot Dysregul. 2023;10(1):11.
316. Salmon AP, Nicol K, Kaess M, Jovev M, Betts JK, Chanen AM. Associations of state or trait dissociation with severity of psychopathology in young people with borderline personality disorder. Borderline Personal Disord Emot Dysregul. 2023;10(1):20.
317. Krause-Utz A, Cackowski S, Daffner S, Sobanski E, Plichta MM, Bohus M, et al. Delay discounting and response disinhibition under acute experimental stress in women with borderline personality disorder and adult attention deficit hyperactivity disorder. Psychol Med. 2016;46(15):3137–49.

318. Ludäscher P, Bohus M, Lieb K, Philipsen A, Jochims A, Schmahl C. Elevated pain thresholds correlate with dissociation and aversive arousal in patients with borderline personality disorder. Psychiatry Res. 2007;149(1–3):291–6.
319. Sommer JL, Blaney C, Mota N, Bilevicius E, Beatie B, Kilborn K, et al. Dissociation as a transdiagnostic indicator of self-injurious behavior and suicide attempts: a focus on posttraumatic stress disorder and borderline personality disorder. J Trauma Stress. 2021;34(6):1149–58.
320. Klonsky ED, Muehlenkamp JJ. Self-injury: a research review for the practitioner. J Clin Psychol. 2007;63(11):1045–56.
321. Kleindienst N, Bohus M, Ludäscher P, Limberger MF, Kuenkele K, Ebner-Priemer UW, et al. Motives for nonsuicidal self-injury among women with borderline personality disorder. J Nervous Ment Dis. 2008;196(3):230–6.
322. Bertsch K, Göhre I, Cottin M, Zettl M, Wienrich C, Back SN. Traumatic childhood experiences and personality functioning: effect of body connection in a cross-sectional German and Chilean sample. Borderline Personal Disord Emot Dysregul. 2024;11(1):20.
323. Löffler A, Kleindienst N, Neukel C, Bekrater-Bodmann R, Flor H. Pleasant touch perception in borderline personality disorder and its relationship with disturbed body representation. Bord Personal Disord Emot Dysregul. 2022;9(1):3.
324. McKinnon MC, Boyd JE, Frewen PA, Lanius UF, Jetly R, Richardson JD, et al. A review of the relation between dissociation, memory, executive functioning and social cognition in military members and civilians with neuropsychiatric conditions. Neuropsychologia. 2016;90:210–34.
325. Haaland VØ, Landrø NI. Pathological dissociation and neuropsychological functioning in borderline personality disorder. Acta Psychiatr Scand. 2009;119(5):383–92.
326. Stevens A, Burkhardt M, Hautzinger M, Schwarz J, Unckel C. Borderline personality disorder: impaired visual perception and working memory. Psychiatry Res. 2004;125(3):257–67.
327. De Ruiter MB, Phaf RH, Elzinga BM, Dyck RV. Dissociative style and individual differences in verbal working memory span. Conscious Cogn. 2004;13(4):821–8.
328. Olsen SA, Beck JG. The effects of dissociation on information processing for analogue trauma and neutral stimuli: a laboratory study. J Anxiety Disord. 2012;26(1):225–32.
329. Amrhein C, Hengmith S, Maragkos M, Hennig-Fast K. Neuropsychological characteristics of highly dissociative healthy individuals. J Trauma Dissociation. 2008;9(4):525–42.

330. Elzinga BM, Ardon AM, Heijnis MK, De Ruiter MB, Van Dyck R, Veltman DJ. Neural correlates of enhanced working-memory performance in dissociative disorder: a functional MRI study. Psychol Med. 2007;37(2):235–45.
331. Dorahy MJ, Middleton W, Irwin HJ. Investigating cognitive inhibition in dissociative identity disorder compared to depression, posttraumatic stress disorder and psychosis. J Trauma Dissociation. 2004;5(4):93–110.
332. Dorahy MJ, McCusker CG, Loewenstein RJ, Colbert K, Mulholland C. Cognitive inhibition and interference in dissociative identity disorder: the effects of anxiety on specific executive functions. Behav Res Ther. 2006;44(5):749–64.
333. Krause-Utz A, Elzinga BM, Oei NYL, Spinhoven P, Bohus M, Schmahl C. Susceptibility to distraction by social cues in borderline personality disorder. Psychopathology. 2014;47(3):148–57.
334. Krause-Utz A, Oei NYL, Niedtfeld I, Bohus M, Spinhoven P, Schmahl C, et al. Influence of emotional distraction on working memory performance in borderline personality disorder. Psychol Med. 2012;42(10):2181–92.
335. Krause-Utz A, Saygin M, Podbylska M, Chatzaki E, La Rosa B, Lis S. Interpersonal emotion regulation, borderline personality disorder symptoms, and working memory during socio-affective distraction. Personal Disord Theory Res Treat. 2025;2025:1.
336. Huntjens RJC, Verschuere B, McNally RJ. Inter-identity autobiographical amnesia in patients with dissociative identity disorder. PLoS ONE. 2012;7(7):e40580.
337. Huntjens RJC, Postma A, Peters ML, Woertman L, van der Hart O. Interidentity amnesia for neutral, episodic information in dissociative identity disorder. J Abnorm Psychol. 2003;112(2):290–7.
338. Dorahy MJ. Dissociative identity disorder and memory dysfunction: the current state of experimental research and its future directions. Clin Psychol Rev. 2001;21(5):771–95.
339. Dimitrova LI, Lawrence AJ, Vissia EM, Chalavi S, Kakouris AF, Veltman DJ, et al. Inter-identity amnesia in dissociative identity disorder resolved: a behavioural and neurobiological study. J Psychiatr Res. 2024;174:220–9.
340. Brewin CR, Ma BYT, Colson J. Effects of experimentally induced dissociation on attention and memory. Conscious Cogn. 2013;22(1):315–23.
341. Paret C, Hoesterey S, Kleindienst N, Schmahl C. Associations of emotional arousal, dissociation and symptom severity with operant conditioning in borderline personality disorder. Psychiatry Res. 2016;244:194–201.
342. Danböck SK, Liedlgruber M, Franke LK, Miedl SF, Hettegger SE, Weber RC, et al. Acute dissociation as part of the defense cascade: associations with behavioral, autonomic, and experiential threat responses in posttraumatic stress disorder. J Psychopathol Clin Sci. 2024;133(1):76–89.

343. Lanius RA, Boyd JE, McKinnon MC, Nicholson AA, Frewen P, Vermetten E, et al. A review of the neurobiological basis of trauma-related dissociation and its relation to cannabinoid- and opioid-mediated stress response: a transdiagnostic, translational approach. Curr Psychiatry Rep. 2018;20(12):118.
344. Sierra M, Senior C, Dalton J, McDonough M, Bond A, Phillips ML, et al. Autonomic response in depersonalization disorder. Arch Gen Psychiatry. 2002;59(9):833–8.
345. Sierra M, Berrios GE. Depersonalization: neurobiological perspectives. Biol Psychiat. 1998;44(9):898–908.
346. Whalen PJ, Kagan J, Cook RG, Davis FC, Kim H, Polis S, et al. Human amygdala responsivity to masked fearful eye whites. Science. 2004;306(5704):2061.
347. Ochsner KN, Ray RR, Hughes B, McRae K, Cooper JC, Weber J, et al. Bottom-up and top-down processes in emotion generation: common and distinct neural mechanisms. Psychol Sci. 2009;20(11):1322–31.
348. Menon V. Large-scale brain networks and psychopathology: a unifying triple network model. Trends Cogn Sci. 2011;15(10):483–506.
349. de Voogd LD, Hermans EJ. Meta-analytic evidence for downregulation of the amygdala during working memory maintenance. Hum Brain Mapp. 2022;43(9):2951–71.
350. Nicholson AA, Friston KJ, Zeidman P, Harricharan S, McKinnon MC, Densmore M, et al. Dynamic causal modeling in PTSD and its dissociative subtype: bottom-up versus top-down processing within fear and emotion regulation circuitry. Hum Brain Mapp. 2017;38(11):5551–61.
351. Nicholson AA, Densmore M, McKinnon MC, Neufeld RWJ, Frewen PA, Théberge J, et al. Machine learning multivariate pattern analysis predicts classification of posttraumatic stress disorder and its dissociative subtype: a multimodal neuroimaging approach. Psychol Med. 2019;49(12):2049–59.
352. Terpou BA, Harricharan S, McKinnon MC, Frewen P, Jetly R, Lanius RA. The effects of trauma on brain and body: a unifying role for the midbrain periaqueductal gray. J Neurosci Res. 2019;97(9):1110–40.
353. Tursich M, Ros T, Frewen PA, Kluetsch RC, Calhoun VD, Lanius RA. Distinct intrinsic network connectivity patterns of post-traumatic stress disorder symptom clusters. Acta Psychiatr Scand. 2015;132(1):29–38.
354. Schlumpf YR, Nijenhuis ERS, Chalavi S, Weder EV, Zimmermann E, Luechinger R, et al. Dissociative part-dependent biopsychosocial reactions to backward masked angry and neutral faces: an fMRI study of dissociative identity disorder. NeuroImage: Clin. 2013;3:54–64.
355. Reinders AATS, Willemsen ATM, Den Boer JA, Vos HPJ, Veltman DJ, Loewenstein RJ. Opposite brain emotion-regulation patterns in identity states of dissociative identity disorder: a PET study and neurobiological model. Psychiatry Res NeuroImaging. 2014;223(3):236–43.

356. Popkirov S, Flasbeck V, Schlegel U, Juckel G, Brüne M. Childhood trauma and dissociative symptoms predict frontal EEG asymmetry in borderline personality disorder. J Trauma Dissociation. 2019;20(1):32–47.
357. Lotfinia S, Soorgi Z, Mertens Y, Daniels J. Structural and functional brain alterations in psychiatric patients with dissociative experiences: a systematic review of magnetic resonance imaging studies. J Psychiatr Res. 2020;128:5–15.
358. Seitz KI, Sicorello M, Schmitz M, Valencia N, Herpertz SC, Bertsch K, et al. Childhood maltreatment and amygdala response to interpersonal threat in a transdiagnostic adult sample: the role of trait dissociation. Biol Psychiatry Cogn Neurosci Neuroimaging. 2024;9(6):626–34.
359. Von Schröder C, Nkrumah RO, Demirakca T, Ende G, Schmahl C. Dissociative experiences alter resting state functional connectivity after childhood abuse. Sci Rep. 2025;15(1):4095.
360. Schmahl C, Arvastson L, Tamm JA, Bohus M, Abdourahman A, Antonijevic I. Gene Expression Profiles in Relation to Tension and Dissociation in Borderline Personality Disorder. Delprato AM, editor. PLoS ONE. 2013;8(8):e70787.
361. Dimitrova LI, Dean SL, Schlumpf YR, Vissia EM, Nijenhuis ERS, Chatzi V, et al. A neurostructural biomarker of dissociative amnesia: a hippocampal study in dissociative identity disorder. Psychol Med. 2023;53(3):805–13.
362. Mertens YL, Manthey A, Sierk A, Walter H, Daniels JK. Neural correlates of acute post-traumatic dissociation: a functional neuroimaging script-driven imagery study. BJPsych Open. 2022;8(4): e109.
363. Mertens YL, Manthey A, Sierk A, De Jong P, Walter H, Daniels JK. A pharmacological challenge paradigm to assess neural signatures of script-elicited acute dissociation in women with post-traumatic stress disorder. BJPsych Open. 2023;9(3): e78.
364. Herpertz SC, Dietrich T, Werth U, Qunaibi M, Lukas G, Schuerkens A, et al. Affect regulation in borderline personality disorder: experimental findings from psychophysiology and functional neuroimaging. Acta Neuropsychiatr. 2002;14(2):71–5.
365. Ebner-Priemer UW, Badeck S, Beckmann C, Wagner A, Feige B, Weiss I, et al. Affective dysregulation and dissociative experience in female patients with borderline personality disorder: a startle response study. J Psychiatr Res. 2005;39(1):85–92.
366. Krause-Utz A, Walther JC, Lis S, Schmahl C, Bohus M. Heart rate variability during a cognitive reappraisal task in female patients with borderline personality disorder: the role of comorbid posttraumatic stress disorder and dissociation. Psychol Med. 2019;49(11):1810–21.

367. Koenig J, Brunner R, Parzer P, Resch F, Kaess M. The physiological orienting response in female adolescents with borderline personality disorder. Prog Neuropsychopharmacol Biol Psychiatry. 2018;86:287–93.
368. Barnow S, Limberg A, Stopsack M, Spitzer C, Grabe HJ, Freyberger HJ, et al. Dissociation and emotion regulation in borderline personality disorder. Psychol Med. 2012;42(4):783–94.
369. Haris EM, Bryant RA, Williamson T, Korgaonkar MS. Functional connectivity of amygdala subnuclei in PTSD: a narrative review. Mol Psychiatry. 2023;28(9):3581–94.
370. Fitzpatrick S, Liebman RE, Monson CM. The borderline interpersonal-affective systems (BIAS) model: Extending understanding of the interpersonal context of borderline personality disorder. Clin Psychol Rev. 2021;84:101983.
371. Arntz A, Genderen H. Schema therapy for borderline personality disorder [Internet]. 1st ed. Wiley; 2020 [cited 2025 Jan 29]. Available from: https://doi.org/10.1002/9781119101161.
372. Fitzpatrick S, Dixon-Gordon KL, Turner CJ, Chen SX, Chapman A. Emotion dysregulation in personality disorders. Curr Psychiatry Rep. 2023;25(5):223–31.
373. Sicorello M, Schmahl C. Emotion dysregulation in borderline personality disorder: a fronto-limbic imbalance? Current Opinion in Psychology. Submitted.
374. Sorgi-Wilson KM, McCloskey MS. Emotion regulation strategies among individuals with borderline personality disorder relative to other groups: A review. Clin Psychology and Psychoth. 2022;2022, cpp.2738.
375. Carpenter RW, Hepp J, Trull TJ. Pain before, during, and after nonsuicidal self-injury: findings from a large web study. J Psychopathol Clin Sci. 2023;132(8):984–95.
376. Ludäscher P, Valerius G, Stiglmayr C, Mauchnik J, Lanius RA, Bohus M, et al. Pain sensitivity and neural processing during dissociative states in patients with borderline personality disorder with and without comorbid posttraumatic stress disorder: a pilot study. JPN. 2010;35(3):177–84.
377. Colle L, Hilviu D, Rossi R, Garbarini F, Fossataro C. Self-harming and sense of agency in patients with borderline personality disorder. Front Psychiatry. 2020;11:449.
378. Polskaya NA, Melnikova MA. Dissociation, trauma and self-harm. Counseling Psychol Psychotherapy. 2020;28(1):25–48.
379. Wilkinson-Ryan T. Identity disturbance in borderline personality disorder: an empirical investigation. Am J Psychiatry. 2000;157(4):528–41.
380. Santangelo PS, Reinhard I, Koudela-Hamila S, Bohus M, Holtmann J, Eid M, et al. The temporal interplay of self-esteem instability and affective

instability in borderline personality disorder patients' everyday lives. J Abnorm Psychol. 2017;126(8):1057–65.
381. Winter D, Koplin K, Lis S. Can't stand the look in the mirror? Self-awareness avoidance in borderline personality disorder. Borderline Personal Disorder Emot Dysregul. 2015;2:13.
382. Thome J, Liebke L, Bungert M, Schmahl C, Domes G, Bohus M, et al. Confidence in facial emotion recognition in borderline personality disorder. Personal Disord. 2016;7(2):159–68.
383. Liebke L, Bungert M, Thome J, Hauschild S, Gescher DM, Schmahl C, et al. Loneliness, social networks, and social functioning in borderline personality disorder. Personal Disord. 2017;8(4):349–56.
384. Lis S, Bohus M. Social interaction in borderline personality disorder. Curr Psychiatry Rep. 2013;15(2):338.
385. Berenson KR, Gregory WE, Glaser E, Romirowsky A, Rafaeli E, Yang X, et al. Impulsivity, rejection sensitivity, and reactions to stressors in borderline personality disorder. Cogn Ther Res. 2016;40(4):510–21.
386. Agrawal HR, Gunderson J, Holmes BM, Lyons-Ruth K. Attachment studies with borderline patients: a review. Harv Rev Psychiatry. 2004;12(2):94–104.
387. Bertsch K, Krauch M, Roelofs K, Cackowski S, Herpertz SC, Volman I. Out of control? Acting out anger is associated with deficient prefrontal emotional action control in male patients with borderline personality disorder. Neuropharmacology. 2019;156: 107463.
388. Bertsch K, Back S, Flechsenhar A, Neukel C, Krauch M, Spieß K, et al. Don't make me angry: frustration-induced anger and its link to aggression in women with borderline personality disorder. Front Psychiatry. 2021;12: 695062.
389. Cackowski S, Krause-Utz A, Van Eijk J, Klohr K, Daffner S, Sobanski E, et al. Anger and aggression in borderline personality disorder and attention deficit hyperactivity disorder—Does stress matter? Bord Personal Disord Emot Dysregul. 2017;4(1):6.
390. Cackowski S, Reitz AC, Ende G, Kleindienst N, Bohus M, Schmahl C, et al. Impact of stress on different components of impulsivity in borderline personality disorder. Psychol Med. 2014;44(15):3329–40.
391. Krause-Utz A, Sobanski E, Alm B, Valerius G, Kleindienst N, Bohus M, et al. Impulsivity in relation to stress in patients with borderline personality disorder with and without co-occurring attention-deficit/hyperactivity disorder: an exploratory study. J Nervous Ment Dis. 2013;201(2):116–23.
392. Kleindienst N, Vonderlin R, Bohus M, Lis S. Childhood adversity and borderline personality disorder. Analyses complementing the meta-analysis by Porter et al. (2020). Acta Psychiatr Scand. 2021;143(2):183–4.

393. Schulze A, Cloos L, Zdravkovic M, Lis S, Krause-Utz A. On the interplay of borderline personality features, childhood trauma severity, attachment types, and social support. Borderline Personal Disord Emot Dysregul. 2022;9(1):35.
394. Miljkovitch R, Deborde AS, Bernier A, Corcos M, Speranza M, Pham-Scottez A. Borderline personality disorder in adolescence as a generalization of disorganized attachment. Front Psychol. 2018;9:1962.
395. Lyons-Ruth K, Bureau JF, Holmes B, Easterbrooks A, Brooks NH. Borderline symptoms and suicidality/self-injury in late adolescence: prospectively observed relationship correlates in infancy and childhood. Psychiatry Res. 2013;206(2–3):273–81.
396. Crowell SE, Beauchaine TP, Linehan MM. A biosocial developmental model of borderline personality: elaborating and extending linehan's theory. Psychol Bull. 2009;135(3):495–510.
397. Zanarini MC, Martinho E, Temes CM, Glass IV, Aguirre BA, Goodman M, et al. Dissociative experiences of adolescents with borderline personality disorder: description and prediction. Bord Personal Disord Emot Dysregul. 2023;10(1):9.
398. Reichborn-Kjennerud T, Ystrom E, Neale MC, Aggen SH, Mazzeo SE, Knudsen GP, et al. Structure of genetic and environmental risk factors for symptoms of *DSM-IV* borderline personality disorder. JAMA Psychiat. 2013;70(11):1206.
399. Witt SH, Streit F, Jungkunz M, Frank J, Awasthi S, Reinbold CS, et al. Genome-wide association study of borderline personality disorder reveals genetic overlap with bipolar disorder, major depression and schizophrenia. Transl Psychiatry. 2017;7(6): e1155.
400. Drews E, Fertuck EA, Koenig J, Kaess M, Arntz A. Hypothalamic-pituitary-adrenal axis functioning in borderline personality disorder: a meta-analysis. Neurosci Biobehav Rev. 2019;96:316–34.
401. Thomas N, Gurvich C, Kulkarni J. Borderline personality disorder, trauma, and the hypothalamus-pituitary-adrenal axis. Neuropsychiatr Dis Treat. 2019;15:2601–12.
402. Stanley B, Siever LJ. The interpersonal dimension of borderline personality disorder: toward a neuropeptide model. AJP. 2010;167(1):24–39.
403. Herpertz SC, Schneider I, Schmahl C, Bertsch K. Neurobiological mechanisms mediating emotion dysregulation as targets of change in borderline personality disorder. Psychopathology. 2018;51(2):96–104.
404. Ruocco AC, Carcone D. A neurobiological model of borderline personality disorder: systematic and integrative review. Harv Rev Psychiatry. 2016;24(5):311–29.

405. Cruz-Ausejo L, Rojas-Ortega A, Valdivieso-Jiménez G, Copez-Lonzoy A, Matayoshi A, Pacheco-Mendoza J, et al. A systematic review of neurobiological aspects of borderline personality disorder among adolescent patients. Biomark Neuropsychiatry. 2025;12: 100114.
406. Marceau EM, Meuldijk D, Townsend ML, Solowij N, Grenyer BFS. Biomarker correlates of psychotherapy outcomes in borderline personality disorder: a systematic review. Neurosci Biobehav Rev. 2018;94:166–78.
407. Krause-Utz A, Winter D, Niedtfeld I, Schmahl C. The latest neuroimaging findings in borderline personality disorder. Curr Psychiatry Rep. 2014;16(3):438.
408. Schulze L, Schulze A, Renneberg B, Schmahl C, Niedtfeld I. Neural correlates of affective disturbances: a comparative meta-analysis of negative affect processing in borderline personality disorder, major depressive disorder, and posttraumatic stress disorder. Biol Psychiatry Cogn Neurosci Neuroimaging. 2019;4(3):220–32.
409. Bilek E, Itz ML, Stößel G, Ma R, Berhe O, Clement L, et al. Deficient amygdala habituation to threatening stimuli in borderline personality disorder relates to adverse childhood experiences. Biol Psychiat. 2019;86(12):930–8.
410. Hazlett EA, Zhang J, New AS, Zelmanova Y, Goldstein KE, Haznedar MM, et al. Potentiated amygdala response to repeated emotional pictures in borderline personality disorder. Biol Psychiatry. 2012;72(6):448–56.
411. Schmitgen MM, Niedtfeld I, Schmitt R, Mancke F, Winter D, Schmahl C, et al. Individualized treatment response prediction of dialectical behavior therapy for borderline personality disorder using multimodal magnetic resonance imaging. Brain Behav. 2019;9(9): e01384.
412. Goodman M, Carpenter D, Tang CY, Goldstein KE, Avedon J, Fernandez N, et al. Dialectical behavior therapy alters emotion regulation and amygdala activity in patients with borderline personality disorder. J Psychiatr Res. 2014;57:108–16.
413. Niedtfeld I, Schmitt R, Winter D, Bohus M, Schmahl C, Herpertz SC. Pain-mediated affect regulation is reduced after dialectical behavior therapy in borderline personality disorder: a longitudinal fMRI study. Soc Cogn Affect Neurosci. 2017;12(5):739–47.
414. Niedtfeld I, Schmitt R, Winter D, Bohus M, Schmahl C, Herpertz SC. Pain-mediated affect regulation is reduced after dialectical behavior therapy in borderline personality disorder: a longitudinal fMRI study. Soc Cogn Affect Neurosci. 2017;12(5):739–47.
415. Schmitt R, Winter D, Niedtfeld I, Herpertz SC, Schmahl C. Effects of psychotherapy on neuronal correlates of reappraisal in female patients with borderline personality disorder. Biol Psychiatry Cogn Neurosci Neuroimaging. 2016;1(6):548–57.

416. Paret C, Kluetsch R, Zaehringer J, Ruf M, Demirakca T, Bohus M, et al. Alterations of amygdala-prefrontal connectivity with real-time fMRI neurofeedback in BPD patients. Soc Cogn Affect Neurosci. 2016;11(6):952–60.
417. van Zutphen L, Siep N, Jacob GA, Domes G, Sprenger A, Willenborg B, et al. Impulse control under emotion processing: an fMRI investigation in borderline personality disorder compared to non-patients and cluster-C personality disorder patients. Brain Imaging Behav. 2019;2019:1.
418. Németh N, Mátrai P, Hegyi P, Czéh B, Czopf L, Hussain A, et al. Theory of mind disturbances in borderline personality disorder: a meta-analysis. Psychiatry Res. 2018;270:143–53.
419. Vegni N, D'Ardia C, Torregiani G. Empathy, mentalization, and theory of mind in borderline personality disorder: possible overlap with autism spectrum disorders. Front Psychol. 2021;12: 626353.
420. Burghardt J, Gradl S, Knopp M, Sprung M. Psychopathology and theory of mind in patients with personality disorders. Bord Personal Disord Emot Dysregul. 2023;10(1):18.
421. Liebke L, Koppe G, Bungert M, Thome J, Hauschild S, Defiebre N, et al. Difficulties with being socially accepted: an experimental study in borderline personality disorder. J Abnorm Psychol. 2018;127(7):670–82.
422. van Schie CC, Chiu CD, Rombouts SARB, Heiser WJ, Elzinga BM. Stuck in a negative me: fMRI study on the role of disturbed self-views in social feedback processing in borderline personality disorder. Psychol Med. 2020;50(4):625–35.
423. Niedtfeld I, Renkewitz F, Mädebach A, Hillmann K, Kleindienst N, Schmahl C, et al. Enhanced memory for negative social information in borderline personality disorder. J Abnorm Psychol. 2020;129(5):480–91.
424. Schulze A, Biermann M, Atanasova K, Unterseher F, Winkler L, Bohus M, et al. Social touch, social isolation, and loneliness in borderline personality disorder during the COVID-19 pandemic. Front Psychiatry. 2022;13: 876413.
425. Kleindienst N, Hauschild S, Liebke L, Thome J, Bertsch K, Hensel S, et al. A negative bias in decoding positive social cues characterizes emotion processing in patients with symptom-remitted borderline personality disorder. Bord Personal Disord Emot Dysregul. 2019;6(1):17.
426. Krueger RF, Derringer J, Markon KE, Watson D, Skodol AE. Initial construction of a maladaptive personality trait model and inventory for DSM-5. Psychol Med. 2012;42(9):1879–90.
427. Bateman A, Campbell C, Luyten P, Fonagy P. A mentalization-based approach to common factors in the treatment of borderline personality disorder. Curr Opin Psychol. 2018;21:44–9.

428. Myrick AC, Webermann AR, Loewenstein RJ, Lanius R, Putnam FW, Brand BL. Six-year follow-up of the treatment of patients with dissociative disorders study*. Eur J Psychotraumatol. 2017;8(1):1344080.
429. Bohus M, Kleindienst N, Hahn C, Müller-Engelmann M, Ludäscher P, Steil R, et al. Dialectical behavior therapy for posttraumatic stress disorder (DBT-PTSD) compared with cognitive processing therapy (CPT) in complex presentations of PTSD in women survivors of childhood abuse: a randomized clinical trial. JAMA Psychiat. 2020;77(12):1235.
430. Harned MS, Korslund KE, Foa EB, Linehan MM. Treating PTSD in suicidal and self-injuring women with borderline personality disorder: development and preliminary evaluation of a Dialectical Behavior Therapy Prolonged Exposure Protocol. Behav Res Ther. 2012;50(6):381–6.
431. Mavranezouli I, Megnin-Viggars O, Daly C, Dias S, Welton NJ, Stockton S, et al. Psychological treatments for post-traumatic stress disorder in adults: a network meta-analysis. Psychol Med. 2020;50(4):542–55.
432. Lewis C, Roberts NP, Andrew M, Starling E, Bisson JI. Psychological therapies for post-traumatic stress disorder in adults: systematic review and meta-analysis. Eur J Psychotraumatol. 2020;11(1):1729633.
433. Schnyder U, Ehlers A, Elbert T, Foa EB, Gersons BPR, Resick PA, et al. Psychotherapies for PTSD: what do they have in common? Eur J Psychotraumatol. 2015;6:28186.
434. Powers MB, Halpern JM, Ferenschak MP, Gillihan SJ, Foa EB. A meta-analytic review of prolonged exposure for posttraumatic stress disorder. Clin Psychol Rev. 2010;30(6):635–41.
435. Wadji DL, Martin-Soelch C, Camos V. Can working memory account for EMDR efficacy in PTSD? BMC Psychol. 2022;10(1):245.
436. Storebø OJ, Stoffers-Winterling JM, Völlm BA, Kongerslev MT, Mattivi JT, Jørgensen MS, et al. Psychological therapies for people with borderline personality disorder. Cochrane Developmental, Psychosocial and Learning Problems Group, editor. Cochrane Database of Systematic Reviews [Internet]. 2020 May 4 [cited 2025 Jan 29];2020(11). Available from: https://doi.org/10.1002/14651858.CD012955.pub2.
437. Foote B, Van Orden K. Adapting dialectical behavior therapy for the treatment of dissociative identity disorder. Am J Psychother. 2016;70(4):343–64.
438. Granato HF, Wilks CR, Miga EM, Korslund KE, Linehan MM. The use of dialectical behavior therapy and prolonged exposure to treat comorbid dissociation and self-harm: the case of a client with borderline personality disorder and posttraumatic stress disorder. J Clin Psychol. 2015;71(8):805–15.
439. Görg N, Priebe K, Böhnke JR, Steil R, Dyer AS, Kleindienst N. Trauma-related emotions and radical acceptance in dialectical behavior therapy for posttraumatic stress disorder after childhood sexual abuse. Bord Personal Disord Emot Dysregul. 2017;4(1):15.

440. Kratzer L, Heinz P, Pfitzer F, Padberg F, Jobst A, Schennach R. Mindfulness and pathological dissociation fully mediate the association of childhood abuse and PTSD symptomatology. Eur J Trauma Dissociation. 2018;2(1):5–10.
441. Sharma T, Sinha VK, Sayeed N. Role of mindfulness in dissociative disorders among adolescents. Indian J Psychiatry. 2016;58(3):326–8.
442. Harned MS, Korslund KE, Linehan MM. A pilot randomized controlled trial of Dialectical Behavior Therapy with and without the Dialectical Behavior Therapy Prolonged Exposure protocol for suicidal and self-injuring women with borderline personality disorder and PTSD. Behav Res Ther. 2014;55:7–17.
443. Bohus M, Kleindienst N, Hahn C, Müller-Engelmann M, Ludäscher P, Steil R, et al. Dialectical behavior therapy for posttraumatic stress disorder (DBT-PTSD) compared with cognitive processing therapy (CPT) in complex presentations of PTSD in women survivors of childhood abuse: a randomized clinical trial. JAMA Psychiat. 2020;77(12):1235–45.
444. Bohus M, Dyer AS, Priebe K, Krüger A, Kleindienst N, Schmahl C, et al. Dialectical behaviour therapy for post-traumatic stress disorder after childhood sexual abuse in patients with and without borderline personality disorder: a randomised controlled trial. Psychother Psychosom. 2013;82(4):221–33.
445. Reyes-Ortega MA, Miranda EM, Fresán A, Vargas AN, Barragán SC, Robles García R, et al. Clinical efficacy of a combined acceptance and commitment therapy, dialectical behavioural therapy, and functional analytic psychotherapy intervention in patients with borderline personality disorder. Psychol Psychother Theory Res Pract. 2020;93(3):474–89.
446. Gilbert P. The origins and nature of compassion focused therapy. Br J Clinic Psychol. 2014;53(1):6–41.
447. Doering S, Hörz S, Rentrop M, Fischer-Kern M, Schuster P, Benecke C, et al. Transference-focused psychotherapy *v.* treatment by community psychotherapists for borderline personality disorder: randomised controlled trial. Br J Psychiatry. 2010;196(5):389–95.
448. Draijer N, Van Zon P. Transference-focused psychotherapy with former child soldiers: meeting the murderous self. J Trauma Dissociation. 2013;14(2):170–83.
449. Van Asselt ADI, Dirksen CD, Arntz A, Giesen-Bloo JH, Van Dyck R, Spinhoven P, et al. Out-patient psychotherapy for borderline personality disorder: cost-effectiveness of schema-focused therapy v transference-focused psychotherapy. Br J Psychiatry. 2008;192(6):450–7.
450. Bachrach N, Rijkeboer MM, Arntz A, Huntjens RJC. Schema therapy for dissociative identity disorder: a case report. Front Psychiatry. 2023;14:1151872.

451. Alberto Barbieri, Federica Visco-Comandini, Alessandra Trianni, Angelo Maria Saliani. A schema therapy approach to complex dissociative disorder in a cross-cultural setting: a single case study. Rivista di Psichiatria [Internet]. 2022 May 1 [cited 2024 Sept. 14];(2022May-June). Available from: https://doi.org/10.1708/3814.37993.
452. Huntjens RJC, Rijkeboer MM, Arntz A. Schema therapy for dissociative identity disorder (DID): rationale and study protocol. Eur J Psychotraumatol. 2019;10(1):1571377.
453. Barlow DH, Farchione TJ, Bullis JR, Gallagher MW, Murray-Latin H, Sauer-Zavala S, et al. The unified protocol for transdiagnostic treatment of emotional disorders compared with diagnosis-specific protocols for anxiety disorders: a randomized clinical trial. JAMA Psychiat. 2017;74(9):875–84.
454. Mohajerin B, Lynn SJ, Bakhtiyari M, Dolatshah B. Evaluating the unified protocol in the treatment of dissociative identify disorder. Cogn Behav Pract. 2020;27(3):270–89.
455. O'Donnell ML, Lau W, Chisholm K, Agathos J, Little J, Terhaag S, et al. A pilot study of the efficacy of the unified protocol for transdiagnostic treatment of emotional disorders in treating posttraumatic psychopathology: a randomized controlled trial. J Trauma Stress. 2021;34(3):563–74.
456. Borderline personality disorder: recognition and management [Internet]. National Institute for Health and Care Guidelines; 2009. Available from: https://www.nice.org.uk/guidance/cg78/resources/2018-surveillance-of-personality-disorders-nice-guidelines-cg77-and-cg78-pdf-6358811143669
457. Hutsebaut J, Debbané M, Sharp C. Designing a range of mentalizing interventions for young people using a clinical staging approach to borderline pathology. Borderline Personal Disorder Emot Dysregul. 2020;7:6.
458. Sharp C, Kerr S, Chanen AM. Early identification and prevention of personality pathology: an AMPD informed model of clinical staging. In: Skodol AE, Oldham JM, editors. The American psychiatric association textbook of personality disorders. Washington, DC: American Psychiatric Association; in press.
459. Iliakis EA, Sonley AKI, Ilagan GS, Choi-Kain LW. Treatment of borderline personality disorder: Is supply adequate to meet public health needs? Psychiatr Serv. 2019;70(9):772–81.
460. Hutsebaut J, Willemsen E, Bachrach N, Van R. Improving access to and effectiveness of mental health care for personality disorders: the guideline-informed treatment for personality disorders (GIT-PD) initiative in the Netherlands. Borderline Personal Disord Emot Dysregul. 2020;7:16.
461. Chanen AM, Berk M, Thompson K. Integrating early intervention for borderline personality disorder and mood disorders. Harv Rev Psychiatry. 2016;24(5):330–41.

462. Gunderson JG. The emergence of a generalist model to meet public health needs for patients with borderline personality disorder. Am J Psychiatry. 2016;173(5):452–8.
463. NHMRC. Clinical practice guideline for the management of borderline personality disorder [Internet]. Canberra: National Health and Medical Research Council; 2013 [cited 2016 Dec 1]. Available from: http://www.nhmrc.gov.au/guidelines/publications/mh25.
464. Linehan MM. Cognitive-behavioral treatment of borderline personality disorder. London: Guilford Press; 1993.
465. Kvarstein EH, Pedersen G, Folmo E, Urnes Ø, Johansen MS, Hummelen B, et al. Mentalization-based treatment or psychodynamic treatment programmes for patients with borderline personality disorder—the impact of clinical severity. Psychol Psychother Theory Res Pract. 2019;92(1):91–111.
466. Horowitz MJ. Psychotherapy for borderline personality: focusing on object relations. AJP. 2006;163(5):944–944.
467. Lanius RA. Trauma-related dissociation and altered states of consciousness: a call for clinical, treatment, and neuroscience research. Eur J Psychotraumatol. 2015;6(1):27905.
468. Zanarini MC, Ruser T, Frankenburg FR, Hennen J. The dissociative experiences of borderline patients. Compr Psychiatry. 2000;41(3):223–7.

Index

A. Krause-Utz, *Dissociation in Borderline Personality Disorder*, https://doi.org/10.1007/978-3-032-06339-7

FSC
www.fsc.org
MIX
Papier | Fördert
gute Waldnutzung
FSC® C083411

Kolibri 360 GmbH
Ferdinand-Jühlke-Straße 7
99095 Erfurt, Deutschland
produktsicherheit@kolibri360.de